TIRED ALL THE TIME

A Doctor's Practical Guide to Finding the Cause & Rebuilding Your Energy

---

Dr Prabhat Das

MD, PhD, FACP

Better Health with Dr Das Series

Hardcover ISBN: 978-1-971672-79-3

Paperback ISBN: 978-1-971672-78-6

eBook ISBN: 978-1-971672-77-9

Printed in the United States of America

Disclaimer

This book is intended solely for educational and informational purposes. It is not meant to replace personal medical advice, diagnosis, or treatment.

Although I am a licensed physician, reading this book does not establish a doctor-patient relationship. Each individual's health condition, medical history, and risk factors are unique. Any medical decision should be made in partnership with your own healthcare professional who understands your specific situation.

Medical science is continually advancing. New research and updated guidelines may lead to changes in recommendations over time.

TABLE OF CONTENTS:

About the Author

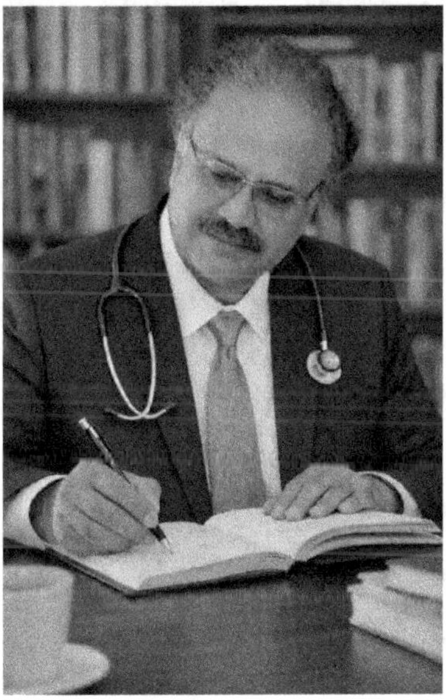

I am Dr Prabhat Das, MD, PhD, FACP. My journey in medicine began in India and, over the past thirty-five years, has continued in the United States, where I have had the privilege of caring for patients across a wide range of medical settings. I am trained in Internal Medicine, Pulmonary Diseases, and Critical Care. For me, medicine has never been just a profession. It has been a lifelong commitment shaped by learning, service, and a deep respect for the trust patients place in their physician.

Over the years, I have had the honor of caring for patients in many different situations. I have seen individuals in my office for routine concerns, treated urgent conditions in busy emergency rooms, managed serious illnesses in the hospital, and cared for critically ill patients in intensive care units. Each setting has taught me something valuable. Each patient has added to my understanding of what it truly means to care for another human being.

But one lesson has stood above all others. Medicine is not only about tests, diagnoses, or treatments. It is about people. It is about listening carefully, understanding fears that are often left unspoken, and guiding patients through uncertainty with clarity and compassion. Again and again, I have seen that what people want most is simple, trustworthy information. They want to understand what is happening in their bodies. They want to feel confident about the decisions they are making for their health and for their families.

These experiences have deeply shaped how I think about health, illness, prevention, and the human side of healing.

That is the reason behind the '**Better Health with Dr Das Series'.** Through these books, I hope to reach individuals I may never meet in person but who are searching for clear and reliable guidance. In today's world, health information is everywhere, yet much of it is confusing, overwhelming, and sometimes misleading. My goal is to cut through that noise and present important medical topics in a way that is simple, practical, and reassuring.

Every page of this series is guided by two foundations: reliable scientific knowledge and decades of real-world clinical experience. I want you, the reader, to feel informed, confident, and empowered. Not overwhelmed. Not confused. But clear about what you can do, step by step, to improve your health.

If even one reader feels less anxious, more informed, or better prepared to take control of their health after reading these books, then this work has served its purpose.

Helping people live healthier, longer, more confident and better-informed lives remains one of the greatest privileges of my life.

CHAPTER 1: Why Am I So Tired?

The Question Many People Hesitate to Ask

"Doctor, I am tired all the time."

I have heard this sentence thousands of times over the years. Sometimes it is said casually. Sometimes it is said with worry. And sometimes it is said quietly, almost apologetically, as if tiredness is too ordinary to deserve attention.

But constant tiredness is not a small thing when it begins to change your life.

It slows your mornings. It makes simple tasks feel heavier. It affects your work, your relationships, your patience, and even your sense of self. It can make you feel older than you are. It can take away the small joys of daily life.

And most importantly, it can leave you confused.

This book begins with a simple but important message:

Tiredness is common, but it should not be ignored.

When Normal Tiredness Becomes a Problem

Everyone feels tired sometimes.

After a long day, poor sleep, emotional stress, illness, or travel, tiredness is expected. In these situations, rest usually helps. A good night's sleep, a quieter day, and proper nourishment can restore your energy.

But constant tiredness is different.

It does not go away with rest.
It follows you through the day.
It is present when you wake up.
It makes you say, "I am functioning, but I am not myself."

That is when tiredness becomes a problem that needs attention.

Tiredness Is a Symptom, Not a Diagnosis

This is one of the most important ideas in this book.

Tiredness is not a disease. It is a signal.

It may come from many different causes:

- Poor sleep
- Stress and emotional strain
- Nutritional deficiencies
- Hormonal imbalance
- Chronic medical conditions
- Medications
- Infections
- Or a combination of several factors

This is why two people with the same complaint may have completely different reasons.

A good doctor does not jump to conclusions. A good doctor listens first.

A Story You May Recognize

Let me tell you about a typical patient.

A woman in her mid-50s comes to the office. She works full time, manages her home, and helps care for her family. For months, she has felt tired.

At first, she ignores it. She blames stress. Then she blames age. She starts drinking more coffee. She tries to push through.

But nothing changes.

She wakes up unrefreshed. By afternoon, she feels drained. She stops doing things she used to enjoy. She becomes irritable. She starts forgetting small things.

Finally, she says, "This is not normal for me."

And she is right.

Her tiredness is real. It may have one cause, or several. But it deserves attention.

If this story feels familiar, you are not alone.

The Most Important Promise of This Book

This book will not give you quick shortcuts or temporary fixes.

It will give you understanding.

By the time you finish this book, you will:

- Understand what your tiredness really means

- Recognize patterns in your symptoms
- Know when to seek medical help
- Learn what actually helps improve energy
- Have a clear, practical plan to move forward

You will move from confusion to clarity.

When You Should Pay Closer Attention

Most tiredness is not dangerous.

But some patterns should not be ignored.

You should take your tiredness seriously if:

- It lasts for several weeks
- It is getting worse
- It affects your daily life
- It is associated with symptoms like weight loss, breathlessness, pain, bleeding, or poor sleep

These are not reasons to panic.

They are reasons to pay attention.

From Guessing to Understanding

Many people try to manage fatigue by guessing.

They drink more coffee.
They take supplements.
They push themselves harder.
They search for answers online.

Sometimes this helps briefly. Often, it does not.

The real solution begins with understanding.

Ask yourself:

- What kind of tiredness do I feel?
- When did it begin?
- What makes it better or worse?
- What has changed in my life or health?

These questions are simple, but powerful.

Doctor's Pearl

Tiredness is not weakness.

It is information.

Your body is trying to tell you something. The goal is not to ignore it or fear it. The goal is to understand it.

Common Mistakes to Avoid

- Ignoring persistent tiredness
- Blaming everything on age
- Using caffeine as a long-term solution
- Taking supplements without knowing the cause
- Avoiding medical evaluation when needed

Chapter Summary

Constant tiredness is common, but it should not be dismissed. It may be caused by lifestyle habits, sleep problems, emotional stress, nutritional deficiencies, hormonal imbalance, chronic disease, or medications.

The right approach is not to guess or ignore, but to observe carefully and understand the cause.

Action Plan

- Write down when your tiredness began
- Notice whether it is improving or worsening
- Identify how it affects your daily life
- Look for associated symptoms
- Review your sleep, routine, and habits
- Seek medical advice if tiredness persists

Looking Ahead

Before we can find the cause of your tiredness, we must understand what you really mean when you say, "I am tired."

In the next chapter, we will break this down clearly. You will learn the difference between fatiguc, sleepiness, weakness, and emotional exhaustion.

This is the step where real understanding begins.

CHAPTER 2: What Do You Really Mean by "Tired"?

One Word, Many Experiences

When a patient tells me, "Doctor, I am tired," I never assume I understand the full picture.

That one word can mean many different things.

For one person, it means they feel sleepy all day.
For another, it means their body feels heavy and slow.
For someone else, it means their mind feels foggy and unfocused.
And for many, it means a deep sense of exhaustion that affects both body and mind.

If we do not define what "tired" really means, we may miss the cause.

This chapter is about clarity. Because the right description often leads to the right diagnosis.

Fatigue vs Sleepiness

This is the most important distinction.

Sleepiness means a tendency to fall asleep.

You may doze off while watching television, sitting quietly, or even during a meeting. You may feel better after a nap. Your eyes feel heavy, and your body is asking for sleep.

Fatigue is different.

Fatigue is a lack of energy. You may not feel sleepy at all. You may lie down and still not fall asleep. Your body feels drained, and even simple tasks require effort.

Many patients say, "I am exhausted, but I cannot sleep."

That is fatigue.

Understanding this difference changes the direction of evaluation. Sleepiness often points toward sleep-related problems. Fatigue may have a broader range of causes.

Fatigue vs Weakness

Weakness is another term that is often confused with fatigue.

Weakness means a loss of muscle strength.

You may find it difficult to lift objects, climb stairs, get up from a chair, or hold things in your hands. The muscles simply do not perform as they should.

Fatigue, on the other hand, is more about low energy.

You may still be able to do the task, but it feels much harder than before.

A fatigued person says, "I can do it, but it takes effort."
A weak person says, "I cannot do it."

This difference is important, because true weakness may suggest a problem with the muscles or nervous system that needs specific evaluation.

Physical Fatigue vs Mental Fatigue

Fatigue is not always the same.

Physical fatigue affects the body.

You may feel heaviness in your muscles. Walking, climbing stairs, or doing routine work feels difficult. Your body tires quickly.

Mental fatigue affects the mind.

You may struggle to concentrate. Reading becomes harder. You may forget things more easily. Decisions feel slow and effortful.

Many people experience both at the same time.

They say, "My body feels tired, and my mind is not clear."

This combination often points toward deeper issues such as poor sleep, stress, or ongoing health problems.

Emotional Fatigue and Burnout

There is another form of tiredness that is often overlooked.

Emotional fatigue.

This is the exhaustion that comes from long-term stress, responsibility, or emotional strain. It is common in people who are constantly giving, managing, and coping without enough rest.

You may feel drained, unmotivated, or disconnected.

You may say, "I just don't have the energy to care anymore."

This is not laziness.

This is burnout.

And it affects both the mind and the body.

Post-Exertional Fatigue

Some people notice a different pattern.

They feel relatively okay at rest, but after physical or mental activity, their symptoms worsen.

This worsening may not happen immediately. It may come hours later or even the next day.

They often say, "If I do too much today, I feel worse tomorrow."

This pattern is important.

It tells us that the body is not recovering normally after exertion. It requires a careful and gradual approach rather than pushing harder.

WHAT IS TIREDNESS?

Tiredness is a feeling of physical, mental, or emotional exhaustion that reduces your energy and ability to function normally.

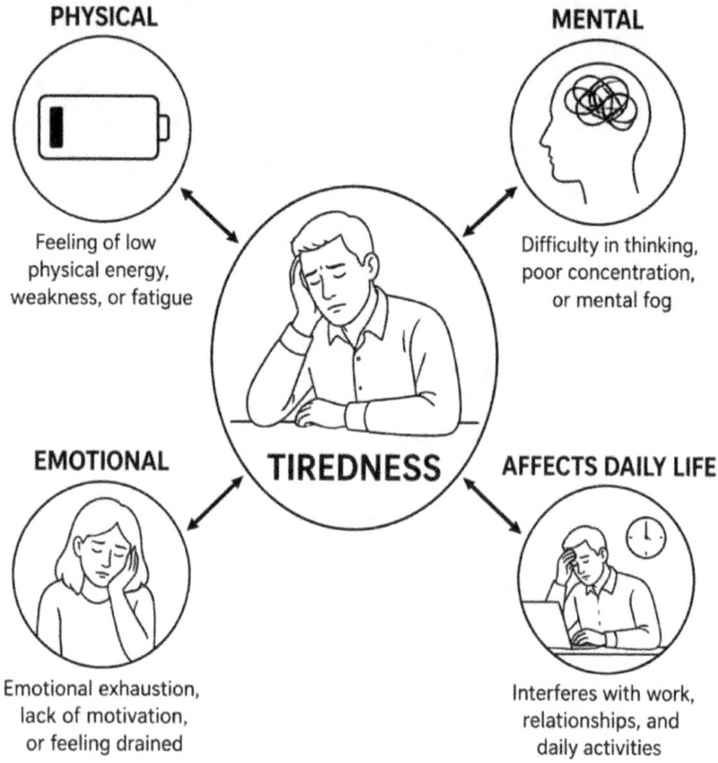

Tiredness is not just feeling sleepy.
It is your body's signal that something may be out of balance.

Why This Distinction Matters

If all tiredness is treated the same way, treatment may fail.

A sleepy person may need evaluation for a sleep disorder.
A fatigued person may need evaluation for medical or lifestyle causes.
A weak person may need neurological assessment.
A burned-out person may need emotional recovery.

The correct path depends on the correct understanding.

This is why taking a few extra minutes to describe your symptoms clearly can make a significant difference.

A Simple Way to Describe Your Tiredness

If you are unsure how to explain your symptoms, try this approach:

- Do I feel sleepy or unable to stay awake?
- Do I feel physically drained or low in energy?
- Do my muscles feel weak?
- Do I have trouble thinking clearly?
- Do I feel emotionally exhausted?
- Does activity improve or worsen my condition?

These questions help turn a vague complaint into a clear description.

A Patient Example

Two patients come to the clinic with the same complaint.

"I am tired all the time."

The first patient says, "I fall asleep during the day, and I feel better after a nap."

The second says, "I feel exhausted, but I cannot sleep. My mind is always active."

These are not the same problem.

The first patient may have a sleep disorder.
The second may have insomnia or stress-related fatigue.

The words are the same, but the meaning is different.

Doctor's Pearl

Never stop at the word "tired."

Ask one more question.

"What exactly do you feel?"

That one question often changes everything.

Common Mistakes to Avoid

- Assuming all tiredness means you need more sleep
- Ignoring true muscle weakness
- Dismissing mental fatigue as normal
- Overlooking emotional exhaustion
- Pushing yourself without understanding your pattern

Chapter Summary

“Tiredness” is not a single condition. It may mean sleepiness, fatigue, weakness, mental fog, or emotional exhaustion. Each has different causes and requires a different approach. Clear description of symptoms is the first step toward correct diagnosis and treatment.

Action Plan

- Describe your tiredness in your own words
- Identify whether you feel sleepy, fatigued, weak, or mentally drained
- Observe how rest and activity affect you
- Write down your symptoms clearly
- Share this description with your doctor

Looking Ahead

Now that you understand what tiredness really means, the next step is to understand how your body creates energy.

In the next chapter, we will explore how sleep, oxygen, nutrition, hormones, and daily rhythm work together to keep you active and alert.

This understanding will help you see where your energy may be slipping away.

CHAPTER 3: How Your Body Creates Energy

Energy Is Built by the Whole Body

When people feel tired, they often think first about sleep.

They say, "Maybe I just need more rest."

Sleep is important, but energy is created by much more than sleep alone. Your body depends on oxygen, blood flow, nutrition, hormones, muscles, brain function, and daily rhythm. When these systems work together, you feel alert and capable. When one or more systems struggle, energy begins to fall.

Think of your body as a carefully organized system. It needs fuel, oxygen, repair, movement, and balance. If any part is disturbed, the whole body can feel tired.

Oxygen and Blood Flow

Every cell in the body needs oxygen.

Your lungs bring oxygen in. Your heart pumps blood. Your red blood cells carry oxygen to the brain, muscles, and organs.

If oxygen delivery is reduced, fatigue can appear quickly. This may happen with anemia, heart disease, lung disease, or poor circulation.

A person may notice, "I get tired climbing stairs," or "I cannot walk as far as before."

This kind of tiredness is important because it may be the body's way of saying that oxygen delivery is not keeping up with demand.

Food as Fuel

Food is not just something that fills the stomach. It is the body's fuel.

Carbohydrates provide quick energy. Protein helps maintain muscle and repair tissue. Healthy fats provide longer-lasting energy. Vitamins and minerals support countless chemical processes that help the body function.

But energy depends not only on what you eat, but also on when you eat.

Skipping meals, eating mostly sugary foods, or depending on coffee instead of real food can create energy swings. You may feel briefly alert, then suddenly drained.

Steady nourishment creates steadier energy.

Blood Sugar Balance

Blood sugar plays a major role in how energetic you feel.

If blood sugar is too high, the body may not use it properly. If it drops too low, the brain and muscles may not get enough fuel.

Both can cause tiredness.

Some people feel tired after large meals. Others feel weak or shaky between meals. These patterns may provide useful clues.

Balanced meals, regular timing, and proper medical care when needed can help stabilize energy.

Hormones and Metabolism

Hormones are powerful chemical messengers.

Thyroid hormone affects the speed of metabolism. Insulin affects blood sugar. Cortisol helps the body respond to stress. Other hormones influence sleep, mood, appetite, muscle, and weight.

When hormones are out of balance, fatigue may appear.

An underactive thyroid can make the body feel slow. Diabetes can cause fatigue through high or unstable blood sugar. Menopause can disturb sleep. Long-term stress can affect the body's rhythm and recovery.

Hormones act quietly, but their effects are often felt deeply.

Sleep as the Repair System

Sleep is the body's repair time.

During good sleep, the brain organizes memory, the nervous system settles, muscles recover, and hormones follow their natural rhythm.

But sleep must be restorative.

A person may spend eight hours in bed and still wake up tired if sleep is broken, shallow, poorly timed, or interrupted by breathing problems.

This is why sleep quality matters as much as sleep duration.

The Brain and Mental Energy

The brain is one of the most energy-demanding organs in the body.

It controls alertness, attention, mood, motivation, and decision-making. When the brain is tired, everything feels harder.

Poor sleep, stress, anxiety, depression, pain, medications, and chronic illness can all affect mental energy.

A patient may say, “My body is not the only problem. My mind feels tired too.”

That feeling is real. Mental fatigue can be just as limiting as physical fatigue.

Muscles and Conditioning

Muscles are part of the energy system.

When you move regularly, muscles become more efficient. The heart and lungs also work better with activity. But when you become inactive, muscles lose strength and endurance.

This is called deconditioning.

HOW YOUR BODY CREATES ENERGY

Your body turns the food you eat and the oxygen you breathe into energy that powers every cell.

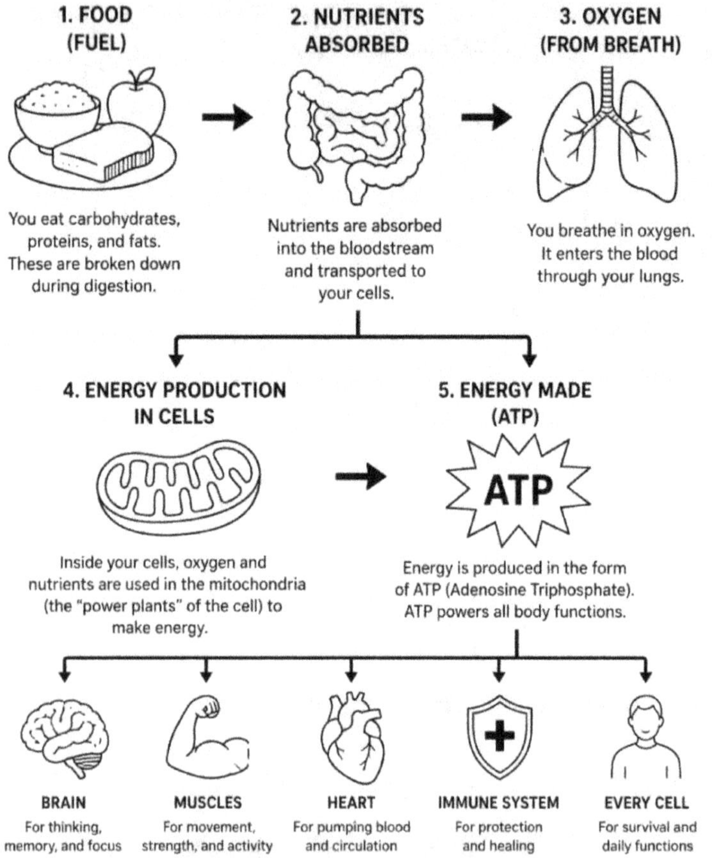

KEY TAKEAWAY

Food + Oxygen → Nutrients reach cells → Energy (ATP) is made → ATP powers your brain, muscles, heart, immunity, and every cell.

A person who moves less becomes tired more easily. Then, because they feel tired, they move even less. This creates a cycle that can slowly shrink daily life.

The answer is not sudden hard exercise. The answer is safe, gradual rebuilding.

Daily Rhythm

The body likes rhythm.

It responds to light, darkness, meals, movement, and regular sleep timing. These daily signals help regulate hormones, temperature, alertness, and rest.

When routine becomes irregular, energy often becomes irregular too.

Late nights, inconsistent wake times, skipped meals, lack of daylight, and too much screen time can all disturb the body's natural rhythm.

A steady routine is not boring to the body. It is reassuring.

When Several Small Problems Add Up

Fatigue often does not come from one single cause.

A person may sleep poorly, skip meals, drink late caffeine, stop exercising, feel stressed, and take a medicine that causes drowsiness. Each factor may be small. Together, they can create major tiredness.

This is why fatigue must be approached broadly.

We must look at the whole person, not just one lab result or one symptom.

A Patient Example

A 61-year-old man comes to the office because he feels tired every day.

He sleeps poorly, wakes up unrefreshed, drinks coffee late in the afternoon, eats irregular meals, has gained weight, and has stopped walking. His blood test also shows mild anemia.

There is not one simple answer. Several factors are draining his energy.

His improvement will also require several steps: better sleep, regular meals, gentle movement, medical evaluation, and treatment of anemia.

This is real-life medicine.

Doctor's Pearl

Energy is built, not borrowed.

You can borrow energy from caffeine or stress for a short time. But lasting energy comes from restoring the systems that support the body every day.

Common Mistakes to Avoid

- Thinking energy depends only on sleep
- Ignoring diet, hydration, and blood sugar patterns
- Using caffeine as a substitute for recovery

- Stopping activity completely without medical reason
- Starting intense exercise too quickly
- Overlooking stress, mood, and mental fatigue

Chapter Summary

Energy is created by many systems working together. Oxygen, blood flow, nutrition, hormones, sleep, brain function, muscles, and daily rhythm all play important roles. When one system is disturbed, fatigue can develop. When several systems are disturbed together, tiredness may become persistent. Understanding this helps us look for the real cause in a thoughtful and complete way.

Action Plan

- Review your sleep quality, not just your sleep hours
- Notice whether you feel tired after meals, activity, or poor sleep
- Look honestly at your nutrition, hydration, and caffeine use
- Pay attention to your stress level and mental fatigue
- Observe whether your activity level has decreased
- Discuss persistent or worsening fatigue with your doctor

Looking Ahead

Now that you understand how the body creates energy, the next important step is learning when tiredness may be a warning sign.

In the next chapter, we will discuss symptoms that should not be ignored, and when fatigue needs prompt medical attention.

CHAPTER 4: When Tiredness Is a Warning Sign

Most Tiredness Is Not Dangerous, but Some Tiredness Needs Attention

Most tiredness is not an emergency.

Many people feel tired because of poor sleep, stress, overwork, irregular meals, lack of exercise, emotional strain, or common medical problems that can be treated. In many cases, energy improves when the underlying cause is found and corrected.

But sometimes tiredness is the first sign that something more serious is happening.

That is why this chapter is important. The goal is not to frighten you. The goal is to help you recognize when tiredness should not be ignored.

A tired body is often asking for rest. But sometimes, it is asking for medical attention.

A Sudden or Major Change in Energy

One of the most important warning signs is change.

If you have always been active and suddenly feel exhausted without a clear reason, take notice.

If tiredness is gradually worsening over weeks or months, take noticc.

If you find yourself saying, “This is not like me,” listen to that thought.

Your body often gives early warnings before a disease becomes obvious. Fatigue may be one of those early warnings.

Tiredness That Affects Daily Life

Tiredness becomes more concerning when it begins to interfere with normal function.

You may have trouble working, driving, cooking, shopping, walking, concentrating, or caring for your family. You may avoid activities you used to enjoy. You may need more rest after small tasks.

When fatigue begins to shrink your life, it deserves evaluation.

The question is not only, “Am I tired?”

The better question is, “What is this tiredness preventing me from doing?”

Shortness of Breath, Chest Symptoms, or Fainting

Tiredness with shortness of breath should never be brushed aside.

If you become unusually breathless with routine activity, or if you have chest pressure, chest tightness, palpitations, dizziness, or fainting, you should seek medical care promptly.

Some heart and lung problems do not begin with dramatic pain. Sometimes they begin with reduced stamina.

A patient may say, "I just get tired when I walk."

That simple sentence may be an important clue.

Unexplained Weight Loss

Losing weight without trying is another warning sign.

If tiredness comes with poor appetite, weight loss, or a feeling that your body is becoming weaker, it needs attention. The cause may be simple, but it should not be ignored.

Unexplained weight loss can occur with thyroid problems, diabetes, digestive disease, infection, inflammation, depression, cancer, or other chronic illness.

Do not assume it is just stress unless it has been properly evaluated.

Fever, Night Sweats, or Persistent Illness

Fatigue with fever, chills, night sweats, swollen glands, or a lingering sense of illness may suggest infection, inflammation, or another medical condition.

Night sweats are especially important when they are repeated, heavy, or associated with weight loss or fever.

Feeling tired after a short infection is common. But feeling unwell for weeks, especially with fever or night sweats, should be discussed with a clinician.

Bleeding, Black Stools, or Signs of Anemia

Hidden blood loss can quietly drain energy.

If you notice black stools, blood in the stool, vomiting blood, heavy menstrual bleeding, unexplained bruising, or unusual bleeding, seek medical advice.

Anemia can develop slowly. At first, you may only feel tired. Later, you may notice dizziness, shortness of breath with activity, palpitations, pale skin, or weakness.

This is one reason tiredness should not be ignored when bleeding is present.

True Weakness or Neurological Symptoms

There is a difference between feeling tired and being truly weak.

If you suddenly cannot move one side of your body, have trouble speaking, develop facial drooping, become confused, lose balance, have new vision changes, or experience severe headache, this needs urgent attention.

These symptoms may suggest a neurological emergency.

Do not call sudden weakness “just fatigue.”

Severe Mood Symptoms

Tiredness can also be linked with depression, anxiety, grief, burnout, or emotional exhaustion.

But if tiredness comes with hopelessness, thoughts of self-harm, inability to function, severe withdrawal, or feeling unsafe, help is needed immediately.

Mental health symptoms are medical symptoms too. They deserve the same seriousness and compassion.

A Patient Example

A 64-year-old man notices increasing tiredness over three months. At first, he blames age. Then he realizes that walking to the mailbox makes him short of breath. His ankles swell by evening. He now sleeps with two pillows.

This is not ordinary tiredness. This pattern may suggest a heart or lung problem.

Another patient feels tired and notices black stools. She becomes dizzy when standing and short of breath while climbing stairs. This may suggest blood loss and anemia.

In both cases, tiredness is not the final answer. It is the signal that begins the search.

Doctor's Pearl

The seriousness of fatigue is often found in what comes with it.

Fatigue alone may have many explanations. Fatigue with chest symptoms, breathlessness, bleeding, weight loss, fever, fainting, or neurological symptoms deserves prompt attention.

WHEN TIREDNESS IS A WARNING SIGN

Tiredness is common, but persistent or unusual tiredness can be your body's way of telling you that something may be wrong.

Listen to your body.

Do not ignore persistent tiredness.

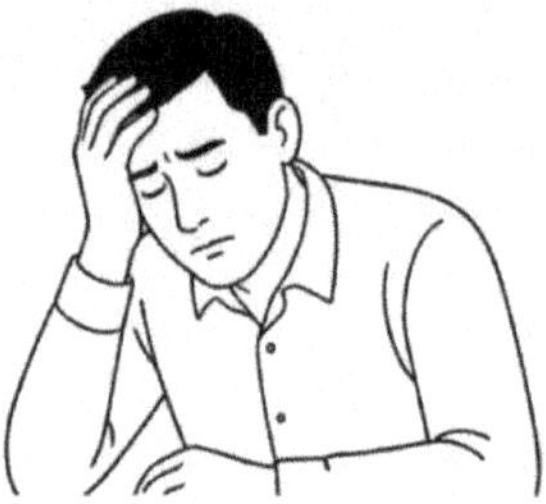

Seek medical attention if tiredness is new, severe, worsening, or affects your daily life.

TIREDNESS MAY BE A WARNING SIGN WHEN IT IS

PERSISTENT
Lasts for weeks or months without a clear reason.

NOT IMPROVED BY REST
Rest or sleep does not make you feel better.

ACCOMPANIED BY OTHER SYMPTOMS
Such as weight loss, fever, shortness of breath, pain, or dizziness.

AFFECTS DAILY FUNCTION
Interferes with work, studies, relationships, or normal activities.

SUDDEN OR SEVERE
Comes on suddenly or is unusually severe.

WITH CHEST PAIN OR PALPITATIONS
May indicate heart problems or other serious conditions.

WITH SHORTNESS OF BREATH
Could be a sign of lung, heart, or blood related problems.

WITH BLEEDING
Such as heavy periods, blood in stool, or vomiting blood.

WITH NEUROLOGICAL SYMPTOMS
Such as confusion, weakness, numbness, or difficulty speaking.

WITH UNEXPLAINED WEIGHT LOSS
May be a sign of chronic illness or serious disease.

KEY TAKEAWAY
Tiredness is not always serious, but when it is persistent, unusual, or accompanied by other symptoms, it deserves medical attention. Early evaluation can help find the cause and prevent complications.

Common Mistakes to Avoid

- Ignoring sudden or worsening fatigue
- Blaming all tiredness on age
- Dismissing shortness of breath as being "out of shape"
- Ignoring black stools or unusual bleeding
- Delaying care when fatigue affects driving or safety
- Calling true weakness "just tiredness"
- Hiding severe mood symptoms from family or your doctor

Chapter Summary

Most tiredness is not dangerous, but certain symptoms should not be ignored. Sudden or worsening fatigue, reduced daily function, chest symptoms, shortness of breath, fainting, unexplained weight loss, fever, night sweats, bleeding, black stools, neurological symptoms, or severe mood symptoms need timely medical attention. Recognizing these warning signs can lead to earlier diagnosis and safer care.

Action Plan

- Notice whether your tiredness is new, worsening, or different from usual
- Pay attention to symptoms that come with fatigue
- Seek prompt care for chest pain, severe breathlessness, fainting, bleeding, or neurological symptoms
- Call your doctor if fatigue lasts several weeks or affects daily life
- Do not rely on caffeine, vitamins, or internet advice when warning signs are present

- Trust your judgment if something feels clearly wrong

Looking Ahead

Now that you know when tiredness may be a warning sign, we can turn to the most common causes seen in everyday life.

In the next chapter, we will look at sleep habits, food, hydration, movement, caffeine, alcohol, stress, and daily routine, the ordinary factors that often have an extraordinary effect on energy.

CHAPTER 5: The Most Common Everyday Causes

Start with the Common Before Searching for the Rare

When people feel tired for weeks or months, their mind often goes to serious possibilities.

They worry about heart disease, cancer, thyroid problems, or some hidden illness. These concerns are understandable, and sometimes medical evaluation is necessary. But in everyday medical practice, many cases of fatigue begin with ordinary factors that slowly disturb the body's rhythm.

Poor sleep. Irregular routine. Skipped meals. Dehydration. Too little movement. Too much caffeine. Alcohol. Stress. Overwork. Caregiving. Burnout.

These may sound simple, but they are not small.

Your body depends on daily habits to create steady energy. When these habits are repeatedly disrupted, fatigue can become persistent.

Poor Sleep Habits

Sleep is the first place to look.

Many people do not sleep enough. Others spend enough time in bed, but their sleep is poor. They may stay on screens late at night, drink caffeine too late, go to bed at different times, or wake frequently.

The body likes rhythm. When sleep is irregular, energy becomes irregular too.

A person may say, "I slept eight hours, but I still feel tired."

That may be because time in bed is not the same as restorative sleep.

Irregular Daily Routine

The body has an internal clock.

It responds to light, darkness, meals, activity, and bedtime. When every day is different, the body struggles to maintain balance.

Late nights, skipped breakfasts, weekend oversleeping, long naps, and inconsistent activity can all affect energy.

A steady routine may sound ordinary, but it can be one of the most powerful medicines for fatigue.

Poor Food Habits

Food should provide steady fuel.

But many people eat in a way that creates energy swings. They skip breakfast, drink coffee instead of eating, eat a heavy lunch, snack on sweets, and then feel drained by afternoon.

The body needs regular nourishment.

Balanced meals with protein, fiber, healthy fats, fruits, vegetables, and whole grains help maintain more stable energy. Highly processed foods and sugary snacks may give a quick lift, but the crash often follows.

Dehydration

Water is easy to overlook.

Even mild dehydration can make a person feel tired, lightheaded, dull, or headachy. Many people drink coffee, tea, or soda but very little plain water.

The goal is not to force excessive water. The goal is to stay reasonably hydrated throughout the day.

Sometimes, a simple habit of drinking water regularly can improve how a person feels.

Lack of Movement

When you are tired, movement feels difficult.

So you move less.

But when you move less, muscles lose strength and stamina. Then walking, climbing stairs, shopping, or cleaning feels harder. This creates a cycle.

Tiredness leads to inactivity.
Inactivity leads to more tiredness.

The way out is not sudden hard exercise. It is gentle, regular movement. Even a short walk can be a beginning.

COMMON CAUSES OF TIREDNESS

Tiredness can have many causes. Often, more than one factor is involved.

1. POOR SLEEP

Not enough sleep, poor sleep quality, or irregular sleep.

2. STRESS & MENTAL HEALTH

Ongoing stress, anxiety, depression, or burnout can drain your energy.

3. POOR NUTRITION & DEHYDRATION

Skipping meals, poor diet, or not drinking enough water can cause fatigue.

4. MEDICAL CONDITIONS

Anemia, diabetes, thyroid problems, heart disease, lung disease, kidney or liver disease, chronic infections, and cancer.

5. MEDICATIONS

Some medicines can cause drowsiness or fatigue as a side effect.

6. HORMONAL CHANGES

Changes in hormones (thyroid problems, menopause, pregnancy, low testosterone) can cause tiredness.

7. INACTIVITY

Lack of physical activity can reduce stamina and increase tiredness.

8. SUBSTANCES

Excess caffeine, alcohol, nicotine, or recreational drugs can lead to fatigue.

9. OTHER FACTORS

Overwork, irregular routine, jet lag, long COVID, or underlying hidden conditions.

KEY TAKEAWAY

Tiredness is a symptom, not a disease.
Finding the cause is the first step to feeling better.
If tiredness persists, consult your doctor.

Too Much Caffeine

Caffeine can help for a short time.

But it can also become a trap.

A person feels tired, drinks coffee late in the day, sleeps poorly at night, wakes tired, and drinks more coffee the next morning. Over time, caffeine is no longer solving the problem. It is helping to continue the cycle.

Coffee is not bad for everyone. But timing matters. For many people, avoiding caffeine in the afternoon or evening can improve sleep and energy.

Alcohol and Late-Night Habits

Alcohol may make you feel relaxed or sleepy, but it can disturb sleep later in the night.

Heavy meals, late snacking, screen use in bed, and irregular bedtime habits can also reduce sleep quality.

A person may believe they slept enough, but the body may not have entered deep, restorative sleep.

Good sleep begins before the head touches the pillow.

Stress, Overwork, and Caregiving

Some tiredness comes from carrying too much for too long.

A person may work all day, care for a spouse, help children, manage finances, cook, clean, worry, and sleep poorly. This is not weakness. This is overload.

Caregivers are especially vulnerable. They often take care of everyone except themselves.

The body eventually speaks through fatigue.

When Everyday Causes and Medical Causes Overlap

It is important to understand that lifestyle causes and medical causes can exist together.

A person may have poor sleep and anemia.
Stress and thyroid disease.
Inactivity and heart disease.
Medication side effects and poor nutrition.

This is why fatigue should be approached with balance. Do not ignore everyday habits. But do not assume habits explain everything.

A Patient Example

A 59-year-old man feels tired every afternoon.

He sleeps at different times each night, drinks coffee at 5 PM, skips breakfast, eats a large lunch, rarely drinks water, and has stopped walking because he feels too tired.

His fatigue is real.

Before assuming something rare, it makes sense to correct the obvious energy drains. If he improves, that is helpful. If he does not, the information still guides the next step.

Doctor's Pearl

Common causes are common for a reason.

Before searching for rare explanations, look carefully at sleep, food, water, movement, caffeine, alcohol, stress, and routine.

Common Mistakes to Avoid

- Ignoring daily habits because they seem too simple
- Using caffeine as a substitute for rest
- Skipping meals and expecting steady energy
- Avoiding all movement because of fatigue
- Drinking alcohol to help sleep
- Blaming yourself instead of looking for patterns
- Delaying medical care if fatigue persists or worsens

Chapter Summary

Many cases of tiredness are linked to everyday causes such as poor sleep, irregular routine, poor nutrition, dehydration, inactivity, excess caffeine, alcohol, overwork, caregiving, and stress. These causes may sound ordinary, but they can strongly affect energy. Correcting them often helps, but persistent or worsening fatigue still deserves medical evaluation.

Action Plan

- Keep a regular wake-up time
- Avoid caffeine late in the day
- Drink water regularly
- Eat balanced meals with protein
- Begin gentle movement if safe
- Reduce alcohol near bedtime
- Create a calm evening routine
- Look honestly at stress, workload, and caregiving responsibilities
- Seek medical advice if fatigue continues despite improving habits

Looking Ahead

Everyday habits can drain energy, but fatigue also affects the body in return.

In the next chapter, we will look at how constant tiredness affects the brain, mood, stamina, sleep, metabolism, relationships, safety, and overall quality of life.

CHAPTER 6: How Constant Tiredness Affects the Whole Body

Tiredness Is Never Just Tiredness

When tiredness continues for weeks or months, it does not stay in one corner of life.

It spreads.

At first, you may only notice that you have less energy. Then your concentration becomes weaker. Your patience becomes shorter. Your activity level drops. Sleep becomes less refreshing. Work feels harder. Family life becomes more strained. Slowly, fatigue begins to touch the whole person.

This is why constant tiredness should not be dismissed as a minor complaint.

It may be invisible to others, but to the person living with it, it can feel heavy and life-changing.

The Brain: Focus, Memory, and Mental Clarity

One of the first places fatigue shows itself is the brain.

A tired brain does not think as clearly. You may read the same paragraph twice. You may forget why you walked into a room. You may lose track of conversations. You may feel slower in making decisions.

Many people describe this as brain fog.

Brain fog is not imagination. It is the experience of a tired nervous system. Poor sleep, stress, pain, depression, anxiety, medications, chronic illness, and inflammation can all affect mental sharpness.

When the brain is tired, even ordinary thinking takes effort.

Mood and Emotional Balance

Fatigue changes mood.

A person who is usually calm may become irritable. A person who is usually cheerful may become quiet and withdrawn. Small problems may feel larger. Patience may disappear quickly.

This can create guilt.

Many people say, "I am not myself."

That sentence is important. Constant tiredness can make a person feel disconnected from their normal personality. It can reduce joy, motivation, and emotional resilience.

The mind and body are closely connected. When the body is exhausted, mood often suffers.

Physical Stamina and Strength

When you are tired, you naturally do less.

You skip walks. You avoid stairs. You postpone chores. You rest more often. This is understandable.

But over time, less activity causes the muscles to lose strength and endurance. The heart and lungs become less efficient with exertion. Simple tasks begin to feel harder.

This is called deconditioning.

It creates a difficult cycle:

Fatigue leads to inactivity.
Inactivity leads to weaker stamina.
Weaker stamina leads to more fatigue.

Breaking this cycle requires gentle, safe, gradual movement.

Sleep and Recovery

Fatigue and sleep often affect each other.

Poor sleep causes tiredness. But constant tiredness can also disturb sleep. A person may nap during the day, feel restless at night, worry about symptoms, or develop an irregular schedule.

The result is another cycle:

Poor sleep leads to fatigue.
Fatigue disrupts routine.
A disrupted routine worsens sleep.

This is why sleep must be addressed carefully in anyone with persistent tiredness.

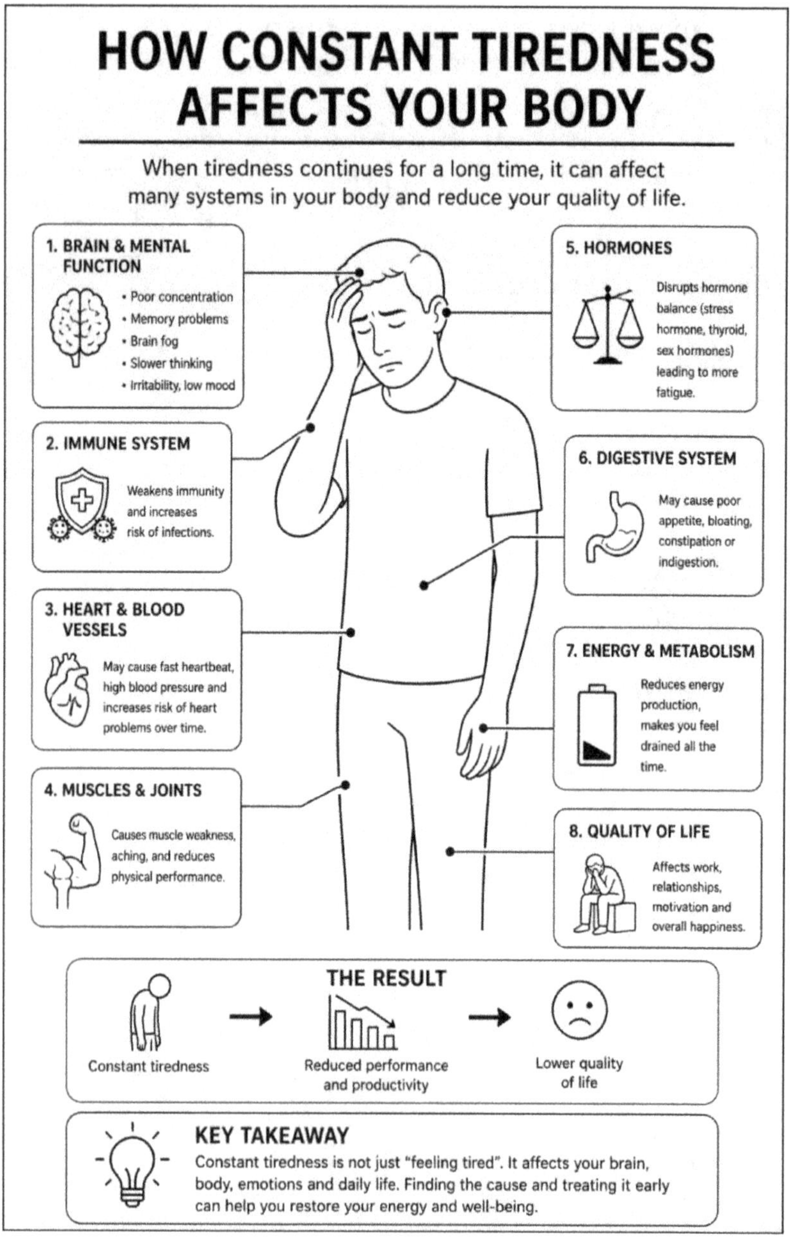
HOW CONSTANT TIREDNESS AFFECTS YOUR BODY
When tiredness continues for a long time, it can affect many systems in your body and reduce your quality of life.
1. BRAIN & MENTAL FUNCTION
• Poor concentration
• Memory problems
• Brain fog
• Slower thinking
• Irritability, low mood
2. IMMUNE SYSTEM
Weakens immunity and increases risk of infections.
3. HEART & BLOOD VESSELS
May cause fast heartbeat, high blood pressure and increases risk of heart problems over time.
4. MUSCLES & JOINTS
Causes muscle weakness, aching, and reduces physical performance.
5. HORMONES
Disrupts hormone balance (stress hormone, thyroid, sex hormones) leading to more fatigue.
6. DIGESTIVE SYSTEM
May cause poor appetite, bloating, constipation or indigestion.
7. ENERGY & METABOLISM
Reduces energy production, makes you feel drained all the time.
8. QUALITY OF LIFE
Affects work, relationships, motivation and overall happiness.
THE RESULT
Constant tiredness
Reduced performance and productivity
Lower quality of life
KEY TAKEAWAY
Constant tiredness is not just "feeling tired". It affects your brain, body, emotions and daily life. Finding the cause and treating it early can help you restore your energy and well-being.

Appetite, Weight, and Metabolism

Fatigue often changes eating habits.

Some people skip meals because they do not have the energy to cook. Others reach for sweets, snacks, or caffeine for quick relief. Some eat late at night because the day has been disorganized.

Activity decreases, and weight may increase. In other people, appetite decreases and weight may fall.

Fatigue can also be connected to metabolic problems such as diabetes, thyroid disease, sleep apnea, or chronic inflammation.

Energy, appetite, weight, and metabolism often move together.

Work, Driving, and Safety

Fatigue can affect safety.

A tired person may make more mistakes, react more slowly, or lose focus. This matters at work, at home, and on the road.

Driving while sleepy or mentally foggy can be dangerous. Operating tools, handling medications, cooking, climbing stairs, or caring for others can also become riskier when fatigue is severe.

This is one reason fatigue deserves respect. It is not only about comfort. It is also about safety.

Relationships and Social Life

Constant tiredness can quietly shrink social life.

A person may cancel plans, avoid visitors, stop calling friends, or become less engaged with family. Loved ones may not fully understand. They may think the person is uninterested, distant, or depressed.

The tired person may feel guilty. Family members may feel confused.

Clear communication helps. Fatigue is not an excuse, but it is an explanation. When people understand that tiredness is real, they can respond with more patience and support.

Independence and Confidence

Persistent fatigue can reduce confidence.

A person may begin to doubt their ability to travel, shop, work, exercise, or attend social events. They may avoid activities because they fear running out of energy.

Over time, life becomes smaller.

One of the goals of treatment is not only to improve energy, but to restore confidence. The person should feel, "I can take steps. I can understand this. I can move forward."

A Patient Example

A 62-year-old woman feels tired for several months.

At first, she only notices that she wants to sit more often. Then she stops walking in the evening. She becomes forgetful at work. She feels irritable with her family. She sleeps poorly, eats irregularly, and begins avoiding social gatherings.

Her fatigue has not affected just one part of her life.

It has affected her brain, mood, body, sleep, food habits, relationships, and confidence.

This is why persistent tiredness deserves a serious and thoughtful approach.

Doctor's Pearl

Fatigue is important not only because of what causes it, but also because of what it causes.

It can slowly reduce movement, confidence, relationships, safety, and quality of life.

Common Mistakes to Avoid

- Thinking fatigue is minor because it is common
- Ignoring brain fog or memory changes
- Dismissing irritability or mood changes
- Becoming completely inactive without medical reason
- Driving when very sleepy
- Letting fatigue isolate you from others
- Delaying evaluation when daily function is affected

Chapter Summary

Constant tiredness can affect the whole body and the whole life. It may impair concentration, memory, mood, physical stamina, sleep, appetite, weight, work performance, safety, relationships, independence, and confidence. Fatigue often creates cycles of inactivity, poor sleep, stress, and reduced function. Recognizing these effects helps explain why persistent tiredness should be addressed early and carefully.

Action Plan

- Notice how tiredness affects your daily life
- Write down changes in memory, mood, sleep, activity, appetite, and relationships
- Avoid driving if you feel very sleepy or unsafe
- Try gentle movement if it is safe for you
- Talk openly with family about how fatigue is affecting you
- Seek medical evaluation if tiredness is persistent, worsening, or limiting normal function

Looking Ahead

Now that we have seen how fatigue affects the whole body, we will look more closely at one of the most common and most treatable causes of tiredness.

In the next chapter, we will discuss sleep problems, including insomnia, sleep apnea, restless legs, and poor sleep rhythm, and how they can quietly steal your energy night after night.

CHAPTER 7: Sleep Problems That Steal Your Energy

When Sleep Does Not Restore You

Sleep should restore the body.

After a good night's sleep, the brain should feel clearer, the body should feel lighter, and the day should feel more manageable. But many people experience something very different.

They go to bed.
They spend enough hours in bed.
They wake up tired.

This is one of the most important clues in evaluating fatigue.

Sleep is not only about how many hours you spend in bed. It is also about quality, depth, timing, and continuity. If sleep is shallow, interrupted, poorly timed, or disturbed by breathing problems, the body may not recover properly.

A person may sleep eight hours and still feel exhausted.

Insomnia: When Sleep Becomes a Struggle

Insomnia can appear in several ways.

Some people cannot fall asleep.
Some wake up repeatedly.

Some wake too early and cannot return to sleep.
Some sleep lightly and wake unrefreshed.

Over time, insomnia becomes more than a nighttime problem. It affects the whole day. A person may feel tired, irritable, foggy, anxious, or less productive.

Insomnia is often linked with stress, pain, anxiety, depression, irregular routine, medications, or poor sleep habits.

The answer is not always a sleeping pill. Often, the first step is to understand why sleep has become difficult.

Sleep Apnea: The Hidden Nighttime Problem

Sleep apnea is one of the most common and important causes of unrefreshing sleep.

In sleep apnea, breathing repeatedly stops or becomes shallow during sleep. The person may not remember waking up, but the body is disturbed again and again through the night.

The result is fragmented sleep.

Common signs include:

- Loud snoring
- Choking or gasping during sleep
- Pauses in breathing noticed by another person
- Morning headaches
- Dry mouth on waking
- Daytime sleepiness
- Poor concentration
- Irritability

Many patients with sleep apnea say, "But I slept all night."

They were in bed all night, but their sleep was not truly restful.

Sleep apnea matters because it affects more than energy. It can be associated with high blood pressure, heart problems, poor concentration, and driving risk. It is also treatable, which makes recognizing it very important.

Restless Legs and Restless Sleep

Some people cannot settle their legs at night.

They feel an uncomfortable urge to move, usually worse in the evening or when lying down. Moving the legs may bring temporary relief, but sleep becomes delayed or interrupted.

Others may not notice the leg movement themselves, but their sleep partner may see frequent kicking or restlessness during the night.

The next day, the person feels tired and does not understand why.

Restless legs and repeated leg movements during sleep can quietly reduce sleep quality.

Circadian Rhythm Problems

Your body has an internal clock.

This clock tells your body when to feel awake and when to feel sleepy. It responds to morning light, darkness, meals, activity, and routine.

When this rhythm is disturbed, sleep may happen at the wrong time or may not feel refreshing.

Common causes include:

- Irregular sleep schedules
- Shift work
- Late-night screen use
- Sleeping late on weekends
- Frequent travel
- Long daytime naps

A person may sleep enough hours, but if the timing is wrong, the sleep may not restore energy well.

The body likes rhythm. Regularity helps sleep become more natural.

Medications, Alcohol, and Sleep Quality

Some medicines can affect sleep.

Certain stimulants may keep a person awake. Some sedating medicines may cause next-day grogginess. Pain medicines, anxiety medicines, allergy medicines, and sleep aids can all affect alertness in different ways.

Alcohol is also misleading.

It may make a person feel sleepy at first, but it can disturb sleep later in the night. The person may wake more often, sleep less deeply, and feel tired the next morning.

If sleep is poor, it is important to review not only bedtime habits, but also medicines, supplements, caffeine, and alcohol.

The Sleep-Fatigue Cycle

Poor sleep causes fatigue.

Fatigue then affects daily habits. A person may nap late, drink more caffeine, exercise less, feel more stressed, and go to bed at irregular times. These habits then worsen sleep.

The cycle continues.

Breaking this cycle often requires small, steady steps:

A regular wake-up time.
Less late caffeine.
A calmer evening routine.
Better light exposure in the morning.
Evaluation for sleep apnea when symptoms suggest it.

Sleep recovery usually improves gradually, not instantly.

How to Know If Sleep Is the Main Problem

Sleep may be contributing to your fatigue if you:

- Wake up unrefreshed most mornings
- Feel sleepy during the day
- Snore loudly

- Wake up choking or gasping
- Have morning headaches
- Have dry mouth on waking
- Fall asleep while reading or watching television
- Feel sleepy while driving
- Struggle to fall asleep or stay asleep
- Have restless legs at night
- Keep an irregular sleep schedule

These signs do not prove a diagnosis, but they strongly suggest that sleep deserves careful attention.

A Patient Example

A 60-year-old man tells his doctor, "I sleep eight hours, but I wake up exhausted."

His wife says he snores loudly and sometimes seems to stop breathing. He wakes with a dry mouth and feels sleepy in the afternoon. He has started nodding off while watching television.

His problem is not lack of time in bed.

His problem may be sleep apnea.

Another patient, a 48-year-old woman, lies awake for two hours every night worrying about work and family. She sleeps lightly, wakes tired, and drinks coffee throughout the day.

Her problem may be insomnia, stress, and a disturbed sleep routine.

Both patients are tired. But the cause is different, so the treatment must be different.

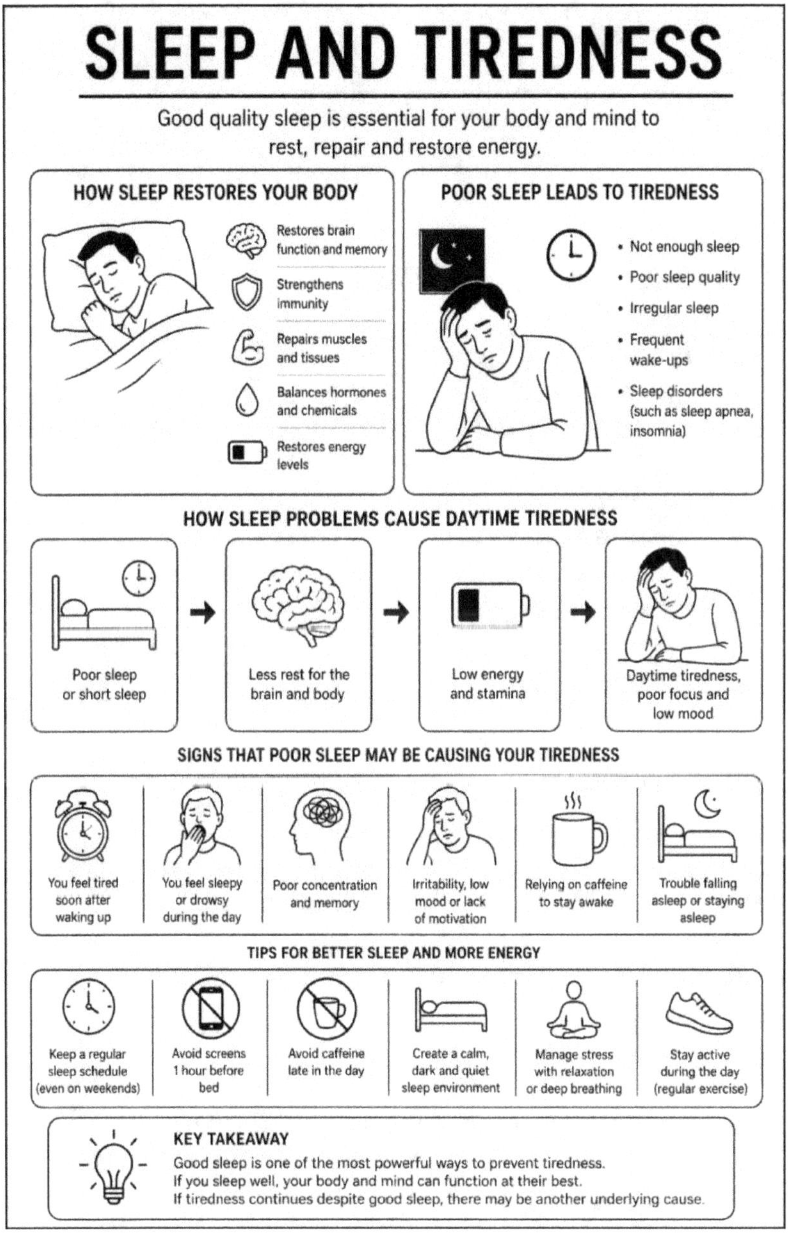
SLEEP AND TIREDNESS
Good quality sleep is essential for your body and mind to rest, repair and restore energy.
HOW SLEEP RESTORES YOUR BODY
Restores brain function and memory
Strengthens immunity
Repairs muscles and tissues
Balances hormones and chemicals
Restores energy levels
POOR SLEEP LEADS TO TIREDNESS
• Not enough sleep
• Poor sleep quality
• Irregular sleep
• Frequent wake-ups
• Sleep disorders (such as sleep apnea, insomnia)
HOW SLEEP PROBLEMS CAUSE DAYTIME TIREDNESS
Poor sleep or short sleep
Less rest for the brain and body
Low energy and stamina
Daytime tiredness, poor focus and low mood
SIGNS THAT POOR SLEEP MAY BE CAUSING YOUR TIREDNESS
You feel tired soon after waking up
You feel sleepy or drowsy during the day
Poor concentration and memory
Irritability, low mood or lack of motivation
Relying on caffeine to stay awake
Trouble falling asleep or staying asleep
TIPS FOR BETTER SLEEP AND MORE ENERGY
Keep a regular sleep schedule (even on weekends)
Avoid screens 1 hour before bed
Avoid caffeine late in the day
Create a calm, dark and quiet sleep environment
Manage stress with relaxation or deep breathing
Stay active during the day (regular exercise)
KEY TAKEAWAY
Good sleep is one of the most powerful ways to prevent tiredness.
If you sleep well, your body and mind can function at their best.
If tiredness continues despite good sleep, there may be another underlying cause.

Doctor's Pearl

Do not judge sleep only by the clock.

Eight hours in bed is not the same as eight hours of good sleep.

Common Mistakes to Avoid

- Ignoring loud snoring with daytime sleepiness
- Using alcohol as a sleep aid
- Taking sleep medicines without understanding the cause
- Drinking caffeine late in the day
- Assuming poor sleep is normal with age
- Ignoring morning headaches or dry mouth
- Driving when sleepy

Chapter Summary

Sleep problems are among the most common causes of constant tiredness. Insomnia, sleep apnea, restless legs, circadian rhythm problems, medicines, alcohol, caffeine, and poor sleep habits can all reduce sleep quality. The number of hours in bed matters, but the quality and timing of sleep matter just as much. Recognizing sleep-related clues can lead to meaningful improvement.

Action Plan

- Keep a sleep diary for one to two weeks
- Record bedtime, wake time, awakenings, naps, caffeine, alcohol, and daytime sleepiness
- Keep a consistent wake-up time
- Avoid caffeine late in the day
- Reduce alcohol near bedtime

- Create a calm evening routine
- Ask your sleep partner about snoring, gasping, or pauses in breathing
- Discuss possible sleep apnea with your doctor if symptoms suggest it

Looking Ahead

Sleep is one of the strongest foundations of energy, but it is not the only one.

In the next chapter, we will look at stress, anxiety, depression, and burnout, and how emotional strain can drain the body just as powerfully as many physical conditions.

CHAPTER 8: Stress, Anxiety, Depression, and Burnout

When the Mind Exhausts the Body

Many people become uncomfortable when a doctor asks about stress, anxiety, or depression.

They may think, "The doctor believes this is all in my head."

That is not true.

Emotional strain can affect the body in very real ways. Stress can disturb sleep, tighten muscles, change appetite, affect hormones, reduce concentration, and drain energy. Anxiety can keep the mind active even when the body needs rest. Depression can make even simple tasks feel heavy.

This fatigue is real. It is not imaginary. It is not weakness.

The mind and body are connected every minute of the day. When one suffers for too long, the other usually feels it.

Stress: Living on High Alert

Stress is the body's response to pressure.

In small amounts, stress can be useful. It helps us focus, act quickly, and solve problems. But when stress continues day after day, the body remains on alert too long.

A person may sleep lightly, wake early, clench the jaw, feel tense, eat poorly, or depend on caffeine. Over time, this constant state of alertness becomes exhausting.

Many patients say, “I am tired, but I cannot relax.”

That sentence tells an important story.

Anxiety: The Mind That Does Not Rest

Anxiety can quietly consume energy.

From the outside, a person may look calm. Inside, the mind may be running all day. Worry moves from one subject to another: health, family, money, work, the future.

This constant inner activity is tiring.

Anxiety may also cause palpitations, stomach discomfort, muscle tension, poor sleep, headaches, and difficulty concentrating. The person may wake up already tired because the mind never truly rested during the night.

Anxiety is not a personality flaw. It is a treatable condition.

Depression: When Energy and Interest Fade

Depression does not always look like crying.

Sometimes it looks like exhaustion.

A person may lose interest in things they once enjoyed. Sleep may increase or decrease. Appetite may change.

Concentration becomes difficult. Motivation fades. Even getting dressed, cooking, or answering a phone call may feel like too much.

Fatigue in depression can be deep and painful.

The person may want to function, but cannot find the strength to begin.

This is not laziness. It is illness, and it deserves proper care.

Burnout: Too Much for Too Long

Burnout develops when demands continue without enough recovery.

It is common in people who carry heavy responsibilities: professionals, caregivers, parents, business owners, healthcare workers, teachers, and anyone who gives more than they receive back.

At first, the person pushes harder.

Then work feels heavier. Patience decreases. Joy disappears. Small tasks feel overwhelming. Eventually, the person feels empty, detached, and exhausted.

Burnout is not cured by one weekend of rest. It often requires a serious reset of workload, boundaries, sleep, support, and expectations.

The Sleep-Stress Cycle

Stress and sleep feed each other.

Stress makes sleep worse. Poor sleep makes stress harder to handle. Then the next day feels heavier, and the night becomes restless again.

This cycle can continue for months.

Breaking it may require small but steady steps: a regular bedtime routine, less evening screen time, quiet breathing, walking, counseling, prayer or meditation if meaningful to the person, journaling, or simply asking for help.

Recovery begins when the body is given permission to come down from high alert.

How Emotional Fatigue Shows Itself

Emotional fatigue may be present when tiredness comes with:

- Constant worry
- Poor sleep
- Irritability
- Loss of interest
- Feeling overwhelmed
- Poor concentration
- Low mood
- Lack of motivation
- Feeling emotionally numb

These symptoms matter.

They are not separate from health. They are part of health.

A Patient Example

A 53-year-old woman comes to the office with fatigue.

Her basic tests are normal. At first, she feels frustrated. She says, “Then why do I feel so bad?”

When we talk further, the story becomes clearer.

She works full time, cares for her elderly father, helps her adult children, sleeps five hours a night, and has not taken a real break in months. She worries constantly and wakes at 3 AM thinking about everything she must do.

Her fatigue is real.

It may not come from anemia or thyroid disease. It may come from chronic stress, poor sleep, emotional overload, and burnout.

Recognizing this is not dismissal. It is diagnosis.

Doctor’s Pearl

Emotional fatigue is still physical fatigue.

The brain is an organ. When it is under strain, the whole body feels it.

Common Mistakes to Avoid

- Thinking stress-related fatigue is “not real”
- Hiding anxiety or depression from your doctor
- Treating burnout only with caffeine and willpower
- Ignoring poor sleep
- Feeling guilty for needing rest

- Waiting until you completely collapse before asking for help

Red Flag Warning

Seek urgent help if tiredness is associated with hopelessness, thoughts of self-harm, severe depression, confusion, substance misuse, or inability to care for yourself.

These symptoms require immediate attention and support.

Chapter Summary

Stress, anxiety, depression, and burnout are common and important causes of tiredness. They affect sleep, appetite, hormones, concentration, mood, and physical energy. Emotional fatigue is not imaginary. It is a real body-mind experience that deserves understanding and proper care. Many people improve when stress is recognized, sleep is restored, support is added, and treatment is provided when needed.

Action Plan

- Ask yourself whether stress has been high for weeks or months
- Notice whether tiredness comes with worry, sadness, irritability, or loss of interest
- Protect small periods of rest each day
- Improve your sleep routine
- Talk honestly with someone you trust
- Discuss persistent anxiety, depression, or burnout with your doctor
- Seek urgent help if you feel unsafe or hopeless

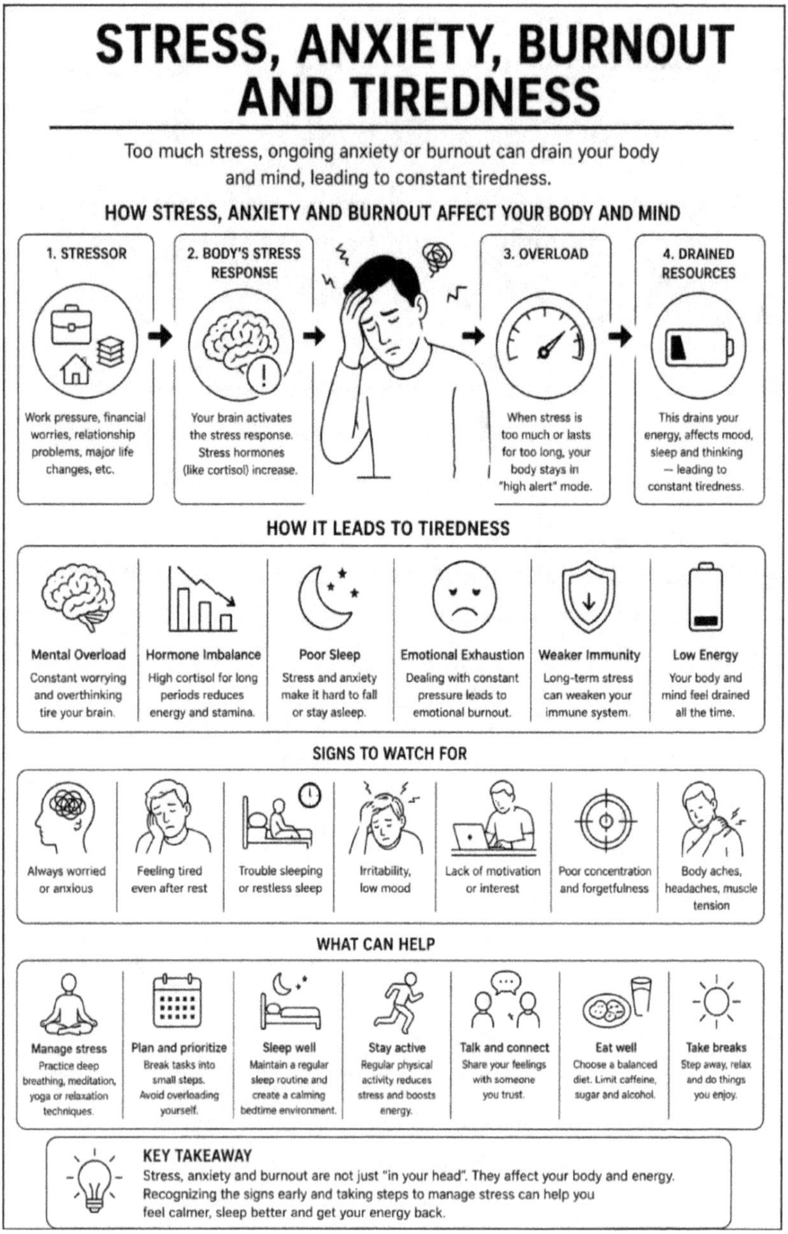
STRESS, ANXIETY, BURNOUT AND TIREDNESS
Too much stress, ongoing anxiety or burnout can drain your body and mind, leading to constant tiredness.
HOW STRESS, ANXIETY AND BURNOUT AFFECT YOUR BODY AND MIND
1. STRESSOR
Work pressure, financial worries, relationship problems, major life changes, etc.
2. BODY'S STRESS RESPONSE
Your brain activates the stress response. Stress hormones (like cortisol) increase.
3. OVERLOAD
When stress is too much or lasts for too long, your body stays in "high alert" mode.
4. DRAINED RESOURCES
This drains your energy, affects mood, sleep and thinking — leading to constant tiredness.
HOW IT LEADS TO TIREDNESS
Mental Overload
Constant worrying and overthinking tire your brain.
Hormone Imbalance
High cortisol for long periods reduces energy and stamina.
Poor Sleep
Stress and anxiety make it hard to fall or stay asleep.
Emotional Exhaustion
Dealing with constant pressure leads to emotional burnout.
Weaker Immunity
Long-term stress can weaken your immune system.
Low Energy
Your body and mind feel drained all the time.
SIGNS TO WATCH FOR
Always worried or anxious
Feeling tired even after rest
Trouble sleeping or restless sleep
Irritability, low mood
Lack of motivation or interest
Poor concentration and forgetfulness
Body aches, headaches, muscle tension
WHAT CAN HELP
Manage stress
Practice deep breathing, meditation, yoga or relaxation techniques.
Plan and prioritize
Break tasks into small steps. Avoid overloading yourself.
Sleep well
Maintain a regular sleep routine and create a calming bedtime environment.
Stay active
Regular physical activity reduces stress and boosts energy.
Talk and connect
Share your feelings with someone you trust.
Eat well
Choose a balanced diet. Limit caffeine, sugar and alcohol.
Take breaks
Step away, relax and do things you enjoy.
KEY TAKEAWAY
Stress, anxiety and burnout are not just "in your head". They affect your body and energy. Recognizing the signs early and taking steps to manage stress can help you feel calmer, sleep better and get your energy back.

Looking Ahead

The mind can drain the body, but the body also needs the right building blocks to create energy.

In the next chapter, we will look at anemia and nutritional deficiencies, including iron, vitamin B12, vitamin D, protein, and other common reasons the body may not have what it needs to function well.

CHAPTER 9: Anemia and Nutritional Deficiencies

When the Body Lacks What It Needs

The body cannot create energy from willpower alone.

It needs oxygen, healthy blood, protein, vitamins, minerals, water, and steady nourishment. When any of these are missing, energy begins to fall.

This type of fatigue often develops slowly. A person may not notice it at first. They simply begin to do less, rest more, and feel older than they are. They may blame stress, age, or a busy life.

But sometimes the real problem is that the body is missing something essential.

Anemia: When Oxygen Delivery Is Reduced

Anemia means the blood does not have enough healthy red blood cells or hemoglobin to carry oxygen properly.

Oxygen is the fuel every cell needs. When the body cannot deliver enough oxygen, fatigue follows.

Common symptoms of anemia may include:

- Tiredness
- Weakness
- Dizziness
- Shortness of breath with activity
- Fast heartbeat

- Headaches
- Pale skin
- Reduced exercise tolerance

Anemia is not a diagnosis by itself. It is a finding. The important question is why anemia is present.

Iron Deficiency

Iron deficiency is one of the most common causes of anemia.

Iron is needed to make hemoglobin. When iron is low, the body cannot carry oxygen efficiently.

Iron deficiency may happen because of:

- Heavy menstrual bleeding
- Blood loss from the stomach or intestines
- Poor iron intake
- Pregnancy
- Poor absorption
- Certain digestive conditions

In adults, especially men and postmenopausal women, iron deficiency should never be ignored. Hidden blood loss must be considered.

This is why taking iron without evaluation is not the best approach. The cause must be understood.

Vitamin B12 Deficiency

Vitamin B12 is needed for healthy blood and healthy nerves.

When B12 is low, fatigue may be accompanied by symptoms that involve the brain and nerves.

These may include:

- Numbness or tingling
- Balance problems
- Memory difficulty
- Poor concentration
- Mood changes
- Weakness
- Sore tongue

B12 deficiency is more common in older adults, strict vegetarians or vegans, people with certain stomach or intestinal problems, and those taking some long-term medications.

This deficiency is important because nerve symptoms can become serious if not recognized and treated.

Vitamin D Deficiency

Vitamin D is important for bone and muscle health.

Low vitamin D may contribute to muscle aches, weakness, and low stamina in some people. It is not the cause of all fatigue, but it may be part of the picture, especially in people with low levels.

Vitamin D should be tested and treated when appropriate. It should not be taken in very high doses without medical guidance.

Protein and Muscle Strength

Protein is often overlooked.

As people get older, recover from illness, eat poorly, or lose appetite, protein intake may fall. When the body does not get enough protein, muscle strength and repair suffer.

This can lead to weakness, slower recovery, and poor stamina.

A person may eat enough calories but still not get enough quality nutrition.

Food quantity and food quality are not the same.

Poor Diet and Energy Swings

Some people do not have a true vitamin deficiency, but their eating pattern still drains energy.

Skipping meals, eating mostly sweets, relying on processed foods, or drinking coffee instead of eating can create unstable energy.

A better pattern is simple:

Regular meals.
Enough protein.
Fruits and vegetables.
Whole grains.
Adequate fluids.
Less dependence on sugar and caffeine.

You do not need a perfect diet. You need a steady one.

ANEMIA AND NUTRITIONAL DEFICIENCIES AND TIREDNESS

Your body needs the right nutrients to make energy and keep you healthy. When these nutrients are low, you may feel tired, weak and unable to function well.

1. ANEMIA – A COMMON CAUSE OF TIREDNESS

Anemia means low levels of hemoglobin or red blood cells. Hemoglobin carries oxygen to your body cells. Low oxygen = low energy.

COMMON CAUSES OF ANEMIA

- Iron deficiency (most common)
- Vitamin B12 deficiency
- Folate (Vitamin B9) deficiency
- Chronic diseases
- Blood loss

2. NUTRITIONAL DEFICIENCIES THAT CAUSE TIREDNESS

Lack of essential nutrients can reduce energy production and affect body functions.

Fe – IRON
Needed for making hemoglobin and carrying oxygen.

B12 – VITAMIN B12
Important for red blood cells and nerve function.

FOLATE (B9)
Helps in red blood cell production and DNA synthesis.

VITAMIN D
Supports energy, immunity and muscle function.

Mg – MAGNESIUM
Helps in energy production and reduces fatigue.

PROTEIN
Essential for tissue repair and steady energy levels.

SIGNS AND SYMPTOMS YOU MAY NOTICE

- Feeling tired all the time
- Weakness, low energy
- Shortness of breath
- Dizziness or light-headedness
- Pale skin, pale nails
- Hair fall

WHAT YOU CAN DO

- Get tested: A simple blood test can detect anemia and nutrient deficiencies.
- Eat a balanced diet rich in iron, vitamins, protein and minerals.
- Take supplements only if prescribed by your doctor.
- Treat the underlying cause (poor diet, blood loss, chronic illness, etc.).

GOOD SOURCES OF KEY NUTRIENTS

- **IRON:** Green leafy vegetables, legumes, beans, lentils, red meat, eggs, jaggery, pumpkin seeds.
- **VITAMIN B12:** Milk, eggs, fish, meat, chicken, fortified cereals.
- **FOLATE (B9):** Leafy greens, lentils, beans, peas, citrus fruits, nuts.
- **VITAMIN D:** Sunlight exposure, fatty fish, egg yolks, fortified foods.
- **MAGNESIUM:** Nuts, seeds, whole grains, legumes, bananas, dark leafy greens.
- **PROTEIN:** Pulses, beans, dairy, eggs, fish, chicken, soy, nuts.

KEY TAKEAWAY

Anemia and nutritional deficiencies are common, treatable causes of tiredness. Eating the right foods, correcting deficiencies and following medical advice can help you feel strong and full of energy again.

Supplements: Helpful When Needed, Not Magic

Supplements can be useful.

Iron helps iron deficiency.
Vitamin B12 helps B12 deficiency.
Vitamin D helps when vitamin D is low.

But supplements are not general energy pills.

Taking many vitamins without knowing the cause of fatigue may delay the right diagnosis. Some supplements can also interact with medicines or cause harm in high doses.

The best treatment is targeted treatment.

A Patient Example

A 47-year-old woman feels tired for months. She assumes it is stress. She begins taking a multivitamin, but nothing improves.

During her visit, she mentions heavy menstrual bleeding and shortness of breath when climbing stairs. Blood tests show iron deficiency anemia.

Her fatigue was not because she was lazy. It was not simply age or stress. Her body could not carry oxygen well because iron was low.

Once the cause is identified, the treatment becomes clearer.

Doctor's Pearl

Do not ask only, “Which vitamin gives me energy?”

Ask, “Is my body missing something important, and why?”

Common Mistakes to Avoid

- Taking iron without medical advice
- Ignoring heavy menstrual bleeding
- Ignoring black stools or blood in the stool
- Assuming all tiredness is caused by vitamin deficiency
- Taking many supplements without a clear reason
- Eating enough calories but too little protein
- Forgetting that deficiencies may be signs of another problem

Chapter Summary

Anemia and nutritional deficiencies are common and treatable causes of fatigue. Iron deficiency can reduce oxygen delivery. Vitamin B12 deficiency can affect blood, nerves, memory, and balance. Vitamin D deficiency may contribute to muscle symptoms in some people. Poor protein intake and irregular eating patterns can also weaken energy. Supplements can help when properly used, but they should be guided by the actual cause.

Action Plan

- Review your diet honestly
- Notice symptoms such as dizziness, shortness of breath, palpitations, numbness, or weakness
- Tell your doctor about heavy bleeding, black stools, poor appetite, or weight loss

- Ask whether blood tests for anemia, iron, B12, or vitamin D are appropriate
- Include protein regularly in meals
- Avoid starting iron or high-dose vitamins without medical guidance
- Focus on steady nourishment, not quick stimulation

Looking Ahead

Nutrition gives the body its building blocks, but hormones guide how the body uses energy.

In the next chapter, we will discuss thyroid disease, blood sugar problems, menopause, testosterone, and other hormonal conditions that can quietly change energy, mood, weight, sleep, and stamina.

CHAPTER 10: Hormones and Energy

Small Changes, Big Effects

Hormones work quietly, but their impact is powerful.

They control how fast your body works, how you use fuel, how you sleep, how you feel, and how your organs stay in balance. When hormones are steady, you rarely notice them. When they are off, the whole body can feel different.

Fatigue is often one of the first signs.

The key is not to chase hormones blindly. The key is to recognize patterns and test thoughtfully.

The Thyroid: Setting the Body's Pace

The thyroid acts like a speed regulator.

When it is underactive, everything slows down. You may feel tired, cold, and mentally sluggish. Weight may increase. Skin may feel dry. Bowel movements may slow. Mood may drop.

When it is overactive, the body runs too fast. You may feel tired but restless. You may have palpitations, heat intolerance, weight loss, tremor, and poor sleep.

In both situations, energy suffers.

Thyroid problems often develop gradually. Many people adapt without realizing what has changed. A simple blood test can help confirm the diagnosis, and treatment is usually effective when needed.

Blood Sugar and Diabetes

Blood sugar is a steady source of fuel for the brain and muscles.

When blood sugar is too high, the body cannot use it well. When it drops too low, the brain and muscles do not receive enough fuel. Both can cause fatigue.

Clues that point toward blood sugar problems include:

- Increased thirst
- Frequent urination
- Blurred vision
- Unintended weight change
- Feeling tired after meals or between meals

Managing blood sugar through diet, activity, and medication when needed often leads to better energy over time.

Menopause and Midlife Hormonal Shifts

Hormonal changes during midlife can affect energy, especially in women.

Hot flashes, night sweats, and sleep disturbance are common. Even if total sleep time seems adequate, repeated awakenings can leave you unrefreshed.

Mood may shift. Weight may change. Daytime fatigue may follow.

Understanding this pattern helps guide treatment. Sometimes simple steps such as improving sleep habits make a difference. In other cases, medical options may be considered after careful evaluation.

Testosterone and Energy in Men

Testosterone levels may decline gradually with age.

Low levels may be considered when fatigue is accompanied by reduced sexual interest, loss of muscle strength, decreased motivation, and low mood.

But fatigue alone does not confirm low testosterone.

Testing should be done carefully, and treatment should be based on both symptoms and results. Hormone therapy is not a general energy treatment and should not be used without clear indication.

Stress Hormones and Daily Rhythm

The body follows a daily rhythm.

Cortisol, a key stress hormone, normally rises in the morning to help you wake up and gradually falls by evening to allow sleep.

Chronic stress, irregular sleep, late-night activity, and shift work can disturb this rhythm.

The result may be difficulty waking in the morning, low daytime energy, and trouble falling asleep at night.

Restoring a regular routine, light exposure in the morning, and calmer evenings can help support a healthier rhythm.

A Word About "Adrenal Fatigue"

You may have heard the term "adrenal fatigue."

It is often used to explain tiredness, brain fog, and low energy.

However, this is not a medically recognized diagnosis.

There is a real condition called adrenal insufficiency, which is uncommon and has specific features that require proper testing and treatment.

Using unproven labels can delay the correct diagnosis and lead to unnecessary supplements.

It is better to focus on clear symptoms, proper evaluation, and evidence-based care.

Recognizing Hormonal Patterns

Hormonal fatigue rarely appears alone.

Look for patterns such as:

- Fatigue with weight gain or weight loss
- Feeling unusually cold or hot
- Changes in sleep

- Changes in appetite or thirst
- Changes in mood or concentration
- Changes in sexual interest or muscle strength

Patterns help guide the next step.

A Patient Example

A 57-year-old woman reports fatigue, weight gain, feeling cold, and slow thinking. Her thyroid test confirms an underactive thyroid. Treatment improves her energy gradually.

A 62-year-old man reports fatigue, increased thirst, and frequent urination. His blood sugar is high. Managing diabetes improves his symptoms.

The symptom is the same. The cause is different.

Doctor's Pearl

Hormones rarely cause fatigue in isolation.

They leave clues. Look for the pattern, not just the symptom.

Common Mistakes to Avoid

- Assuming every tired person has a hormonal problem
- Starting hormone therapy without proper testing
- Relying on internet diagnoses
- Ignoring associated symptoms
- Taking supplements marketed for "hormone balance" without guidance

HORMONES AND FATIGUE

Hormones are chemical messengers that control many body functions. When hormone levels are too high, too low, or out of balance, it can lead to fatigue and low energy.

KEY HORMONES THAT AFFECT ENERGY

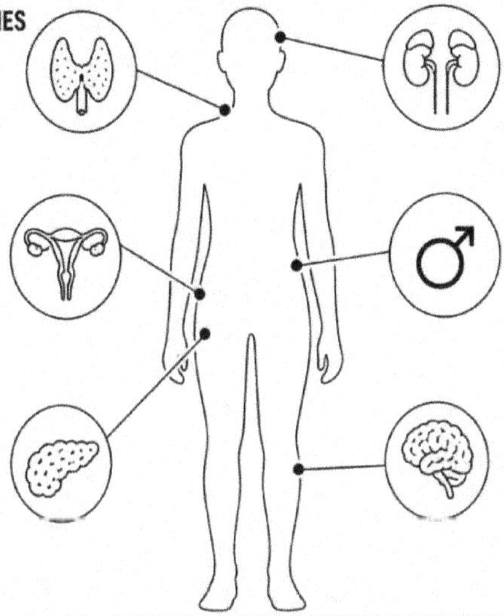

THYROID HORMONES (T3, T4)

Regulate metabolism. Low levels can cause fatigue, weight gain, cold intolerance, and depression.

ESTROGEN & PROGESTERONE

Fluctuations during menstruation, pregnancy, or menopause can cause tiredness, mood changes, and low energy.

INSULIN

Helps regulate blood sugar. Insulin resistance or blood sugar swings can lead to fatigue after meals and low energy.

CORTISOL

The stress hormone. Chronic high or low levels can cause exhaustion, poor sleep, and difficulty concentrating.

TESTOSTERONE

Low levels (in men and women) can cause fatigue, low motivation, reduced muscle strength, and low energy.

GROWTH HORMONE & MELATONIN

Affect sleep quality and recovery. Imbalance can cause poor sleep and daytime fatigue.

SIGNS HORMONES MAY BE CAUSING FATIGUE

- Fatigue despite enough sleep
- Unexplained weight gain or loss
- Brain fog and poor concentration
- Mood swings, irritability, or anxiety
- Irregular or heavy periods
- Trouble sleeping or waking up unrefreshed

COMMON CAUSES OF HORMONAL IMBALANCE

- Chronic stress
- Poor diet and nutrient deficiencies
- Lack of sleep
- Overexercising
- Medical conditions (thyroid disorders, PCOS, diabetes, adrenal fatigue, etc.)
- Aging and hormonal changes

WHAT YOU CAN DO

- Get tested: Blood tests can identify hormonal imbalances.
- Eat a balanced diet with whole foods and enough protein.
- Manage stress with relaxation, breathing, yoga, or meditation.
- Sleep 7–9 hours every night.
- Work with a healthcare professional for proper diagnosis and treatment.

KEY TAKEAWAY

Hormonal imbalances are a common cause of fatigue. Identifying the root cause and restoring balance can help you feel more energized, healthy, and in control.

Chapter Summary

Hormones play a central role in energy. Thyroid disease, blood sugar problems, menopause, and other hormonal changes can affect how you feel. These conditions usually present with patterns of symptoms rather than fatigue alone. Proper evaluation and targeted treatment are essential for recovery.

Action Plan

- Notice associated symptoms such as weight change, temperature sensitivity, sleep disturbance, and appetite changes
- Discuss appropriate testing with your doctor
- Avoid self-treatment with hormone supplements
- Maintain a regular daily routine to support natural hormonal rhythm
- Follow up if symptoms persist or change

Looking Ahead

Hormones are one part of the picture. Many long-term medical conditions can also drain energy slowly and quietly.

In the next chapter, we will look at how heart, lung, kidney, liver, and other chronic diseases can affect stamina, breathing, and daily function.

CHAPTER 11: Chronic Diseases That Quietly Drain Your Energy

When Tiredness Comes from a Deeper Illness

Sometimes tiredness does not come from poor sleep, stress, diet, or routine.

Sometimes it comes from the body working harder than it should.

Many chronic diseases develop slowly. In the beginning, the body adjusts. Symptoms may be mild, vague, or easy to dismiss. A person may not feel "sick." They may simply notice that they cannot do as much as before.

Fatigue may be the first clue.

This does not mean you should become fearful every time you feel tired. Most tiredness is not due to serious disease. But persistent or worsening fatigue deserves careful attention, especially when it comes with other symptoms.

Heart Disease: When the Pump Is Under Strain

The heart supplies blood and oxygen to the entire body.

When the heart is not working efficiently, the muscles and organs may not receive enough blood flow during activity. The result may be tiredness, weakness, shortness of breath, dizziness, or reduced stamina.

Some people expect heart disease to always cause chest pain. But that is not always the case.

Sometimes a person simply says, “I cannot walk as far as I used to,” or “I get tired doing ordinary things.”

Other clues may include swelling of the feet or ankles, breathlessness when lying flat, palpitations, chest pressure, or needing more pillows at night.

A change in exercise tolerance should always be respected.

Lung Disease: When Breathing Takes Too Much Effort

The lungs bring oxygen into the body.

When lung function is reduced, breathing becomes harder work. This may happen with conditions such as COPD, asthma, pulmonary fibrosis, or other lung problems.

A person may feel tired because the body is using extra energy just to breathe.

Common clues include:

- Shortness of breath
- Chronic cough
- Wheezing
- Chest tightness
- Low oxygen levels
- Reduced ability to walk or climb stairs

Some patients do not describe breathlessness clearly. They may simply say, “I get tired quickly.”

That statement may be an important clue.

Kidney Disease: When the Body Cannot Clear Waste Well

The kidneys filter waste, balance fluids, regulate minerals, help control blood pressure, and support red blood cell production.

When kidney function declines, fatigue may develop for several reasons. Waste products may build up. Anemia may occur. Appetite may decrease. Sleep may worsen. Fluid balance may change.

Symptoms may include:

- Tiredness
- Swelling of the legs or feet
- Changes in urination
- Poor appetite
- Nausea
- Itching
- Trouble sleeping

Kidney disease can be quiet for a long time. This is why people with diabetes, high blood pressure, or a family history of kidney disease need regular monitoring.

Liver Disease: When Metabolism Is Disturbed

The liver is one of the body’s busiest organs.

It processes nutrients, handles toxins, makes important proteins, helps with digestion, and supports energy metabolism.

When the liver is not working well, fatigue can be one of the earliest symptoms.

Other clues may include poor appetite, nausea, abdominal swelling, yellowing of the skin or eyes, dark urine, itching, easy bruising, or confusion in more advanced disease.

Fatty liver disease, hepatitis, alcohol-related liver disease, autoimmune liver disease, and cirrhosis can all cause fatigue.

Early liver disease may be silent, so abnormal liver tests or persistent symptoms should not be ignored.

Autoimmune and Inflammatory Conditions

In autoimmune diseases, the immune system mistakenly attacks the body's own tissues.

This can create ongoing inflammation, pain, and fatigue.

Examples include rheumatoid arthritis, lupus, inflammatory bowel disease, multiple sclerosis, and certain thyroid conditions.

Fatigue from inflammation often feels deep and heavy. It may come with joint pain, swelling, morning stiffness, rashes, mouth ulcers, bowel symptoms, fevers, or muscle aches.

A patient may say, "I feel like I have the flu, but it never fully goes away."

That kind of fatigue deserves evaluation.

Cancer and Serious Illness

Most fatigue is not cancer.

This is very important to say clearly.

However, fatigue can sometimes be part of serious illness. The concern becomes stronger when tiredness comes with unexplained weight loss, persistent pain, poor appetite, fever, night sweats, bleeding, or a new lump.

The purpose of evaluation is not to assume the worst. It is to avoid missing something important.

Early attention can make a real difference.

When More Than One Problem Exists

In real life, fatigue often comes from several causes at the same time.

A person may have mild heart disease, poor sleep, diabetes, medication side effects, and low activity. Another may have kidney disease, anemia, and depression. Another may have COPD, poor nutrition, and sleep apnea.

Each factor may contribute a little. Together, they create major fatigue.

This is why a broad, thoughtful approach is needed.

A Patient Example

A 69-year-old man feels tired for several months.

At first, he blames aging. Then he notices that he cannot walk as far as before. His ankles swell by evening. He feels short of breath when climbing stairs and sleeps better with extra pillows.

This pattern may point toward heart disease or heart failure.

Another patient feels tired, itchy, nauseated, and notices changes in urination. This pattern may suggest kidney involvement.

The symptom is the same: tiredness.

But the story behind it is different.

Doctor's Pearl

Chronic disease fatigue often reveals itself through lost function.

Pay attention not only to how tired you feel, but also to what you can no longer do comfortably.

Common Mistakes to Avoid

- Blaming all fatigue on age
- Ignoring reduced walking distance or stamina

- Dismissing shortness of breath as poor fitness without evaluation
- Ignoring swelling of the legs or feet
- Overlooking changes in urination, appetite, or weight
- Assuming normal basic tests explain everything
- Delaying follow-up for known chronic diseases

Chapter Summary

Chronic diseases can quietly drain energy by affecting oxygen delivery, circulation, breathing, waste removal, metabolism, inflammation, sleep, and muscle function. Heart disease, lung disease, kidney disease, liver disease, autoimmune illness, and serious conditions can all cause fatigue. The key is to look for patterns and associated symptoms rather than guessing. Persistent or worsening fatigue should be discussed with a doctor, especially when daily function is changing.

Action Plan

- Notice whether your stamina has changed
- Pay attention to shortness of breath, swelling, cough, pain, itching, weight loss, appetite change, or changes in urination
- Keep regular follow-up for diabetes, high blood pressure, heart disease, lung disease, kidney disease, or liver disease
- Do not stop prescribed medicines without guidance
- Seek prompt medical care if fatigue comes with chest pain, fainting, severe breathlessness, bleeding, confusion, or neurological symptoms
- Tell your doctor how fatigue is affecting your daily function, not just that you feel tired

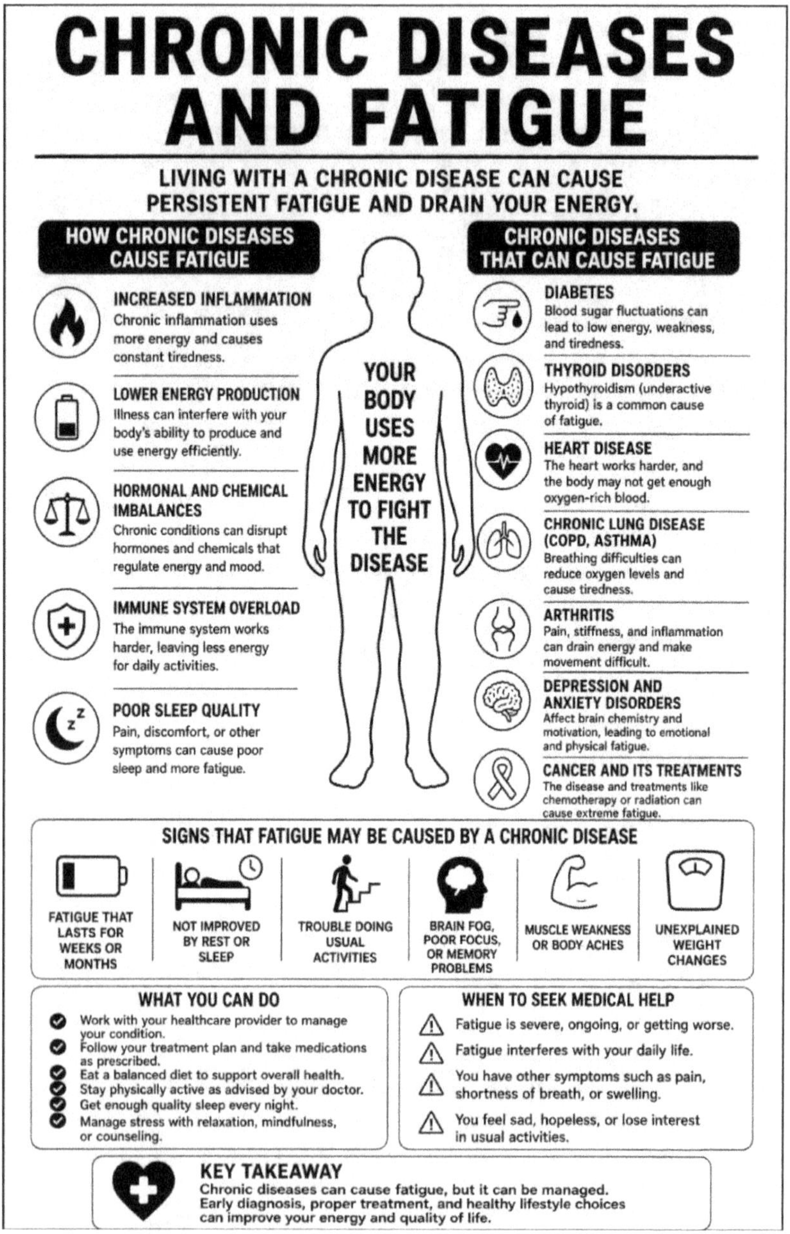

CHRONIC DISEASES AND FATIGUE
LIVING WITH A CHRONIC DISEASE CAN CAUSE PERSISTENT FATIGUE AND DRAIN YOUR ENERGY.
HOW CHRONIC DISEASES CAUSE FATIGUE
INCREASED INFLAMMATION
Chronic inflammation uses more energy and causes constant tiredness.
LOWER ENERGY PRODUCTION
Illness can interfere with your body's ability to produce and use energy efficiently.
HORMONAL AND CHEMICAL IMBALANCES
Chronic conditions can disrupt hormones and chemicals that regulate energy and mood.
IMMUNE SYSTEM OVERLOAD
The immune system works harder, leaving less energy for daily activities.
POOR SLEEP QUALITY
Pain, discomfort, or other symptoms can cause poor sleep and more fatigue.
YOUR BODY USES MORE ENERGY TO FIGHT THE DISEASE
CHRONIC DISEASES THAT CAN CAUSE FATIGUE
DIABETES
Blood sugar fluctuations can lead to low energy, weakness, and tiredness.
THYROID DISORDERS
Hypothyroidism (underactive thyroid) is a common cause of fatigue.
HEART DISEASE
The heart works harder, and the body may not get enough oxygen-rich blood.
CHRONIC LUNG DISEASE (COPD, ASTHMA)
Breathing difficulties can reduce oxygen levels and cause tiredness.
ARTHRITIS
Pain, stiffness, and inflammation can drain energy and make movement difficult.
DEPRESSION AND ANXIETY DISORDERS
Affect brain chemistry and motivation, leading to emotional and physical fatigue.
CANCER AND ITS TREATMENTS
The disease and treatments like chemotherapy or radiation can cause extreme fatigue.
SIGNS THAT FATIGUE MAY BE CAUSED BY A CHRONIC DISEASE
FATIGUE THAT LASTS FOR WEEKS OR MONTHS
NOT IMPROVED BY REST OR SLEEP
TROUBLE DOING USUAL ACTIVITIES
BRAIN FOG, POOR FOCUS, OR MEMORY PROBLEMS
MUSCLE WEAKNESS OR BODY ACHES
UNEXPLAINED WEIGHT CHANGES
WHAT YOU CAN DO
Work with your healthcare provider to manage your condition.
Follow your treatment plan and take medications as prescribed.
Eat a balanced diet to support overall health.
Stay physically active as advised by your doctor.
Get enough quality sleep every night.
Manage stress with relaxation, mindfulness, or counseling.
WHEN TO SEEK MEDICAL HELP
Fatigue is severe, ongoing, or getting worse.
Fatigue interferes with your daily life.
You have other symptoms such as pain, shortness of breath, or swelling.
You feel sad, hopeless, or lose interest in usual activities.
KEY TAKEAWAY
Chronic diseases can cause fatigue, but it can be managed. Early diagnosis, proper treatment, and healthy lifestyle choices can improve your energy and quality of life.

Looking Ahead

Chronic diseases can drain energy slowly, but infections can also leave the body exhausted long after the original illness has passed.

In the next chapter, we will discuss post-illness fatigue, Long COVID, chronic fatigue syndrome, and the important warning sign called post-exertional malaise.

CHAPTER 12: Infections, Long COVID, and Post-Illness Fatigue

When Recovery Takes Longer Than Expected

Most infections follow a familiar path.

You fall sick. You rest. You recover. Life returns to normal.

But sometimes, that last step does not happen.

The fever goes away. The cough improves. The infection seems over. Yet the tiredness remains. Days pass. Weeks pass. Energy does not return.

Patients often say, "I never got my strength back."

This kind of fatigue is real. It is not uncommon. And it deserves attention.

After Common Infections

Even routine infections can leave the body temporarily drained.

After viral illnesses, the immune system takes time to settle. Muscles may feel weak. Sleep may be disturbed. Appetite may change. The body is still recovering, even though the main symptoms are gone.

In most cases, energy returns gradually.

But when fatigue continues longer than expected, especially beyond a few weeks, it should not be ignored.

Long COVID: A New Pattern of Fatigue

One of the most important developments in recent years has been Long COVID.

Some people continue to experience symptoms long after the initial infection has resolved. Fatigue is one of the most common and troubling symptoms.

This fatigue may come with:

- Brain fog
- Poor concentration
- Shortness of breath
- Palpitations
- Poor sleep
- Headaches
- Muscle aches

What makes it different is its unpredictability.

A person may feel relatively well one day and completely drained the next.

This pattern can be frustrating and confusing.

Post-Exertional Malaise

One of the most important features of post-illness fatigue is post-exertional malaise.

This means symptoms worsen after physical or mental effort.

The worsening may not happen immediately. It may appear hours later or even the next day.

Patients often say, "If I do too much today, I feel much worse tomorrow."

This is a key clue.

It changes how recovery should be approached. Pushing harder is not always helpful. In some cases, it can make symptoms worse.

Chronic Fatigue Syndrome (ME/CFS)

Chronic fatigue syndrome, also known as myalgic encephalomyelitis, is a condition where fatigue persists for months and is not relieved by rest.

It is often associated with:

- Post-exertional malaise
- Unrefreshing sleep
- Cognitive difficulties
- Low stamina

This condition is not fully understood, but it is recognized as real and complex.

People with this pattern need careful evaluation and a balanced approach to activity and rest.

Why Does Post-Illness Fatigue Happen?

The exact reasons are still being studied.

Possible factors include:

- Ongoing low-level inflammation
- Changes in the immune system
- Effects on the brain and nervous system
- Disturbances in energy production
- Sleep disruption
- Deconditioning after illness

In many cases, more than one factor is involved.

Understanding this helps explain why recovery may take time.

The Right Approach to Recovery

Recovery from post-illness fatigue is different from recovery from simple tiredness.

Two extremes should be avoided.

Pushing too hard can worsen symptoms.
Doing nothing for too long can weaken the body further.

The goal is balance.

Gradual, paced activity with proper rest is often the safest approach.

Small steps, repeated consistently, help the body rebuild strength.

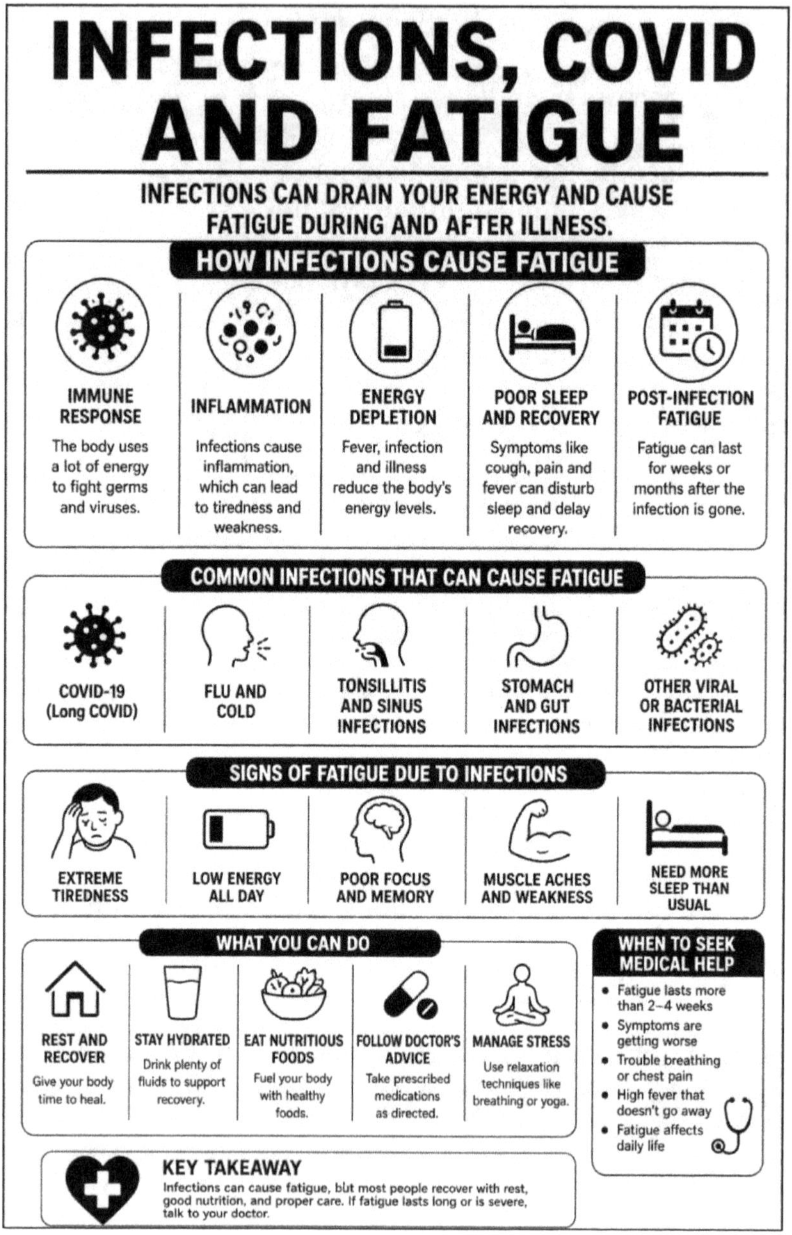
INFECTIONS, COVID AND FATIGUE
INFECTIONS CAN DRAIN YOUR ENERGY AND CAUSE FATIGUE DURING AND AFTER ILLNESS.
HOW INFECTIONS CAUSE FATIGUE
IMMUNE RESPONSE
The body uses a lot of energy to fight germs and viruses.
INFLAMMATION
Infections cause inflammation, which can lead to tiredness and weakness.
ENERGY DEPLETION
Fever, infection and illness reduce the body's energy levels.
POOR SLEEP AND RECOVERY
Symptoms like cough, pain and fever can disturb sleep and delay recovery.
POST-INFECTION FATIGUE
Fatigue can last for weeks or months after the infection is gone.
COMMON INFECTIONS THAT CAN CAUSE FATIGUE
COVID-19 (Long COVID)
FLU AND COLD
TONSILLITIS AND SINUS INFECTIONS
STOMACH AND GUT INFECTIONS
OTHER VIRAL OR BACTERIAL INFECTIONS
SIGNS OF FATIGUE DUE TO INFECTIONS
EXTREME TIREDNESS
LOW ENERGY ALL DAY
POOR FOCUS AND MEMORY
MUSCLE ACHES AND WEAKNESS
NEED MORE SLEEP THAN USUAL
WHAT YOU CAN DO
REST AND RECOVER
Give your body time to heal.
STAY HYDRATED
Drink plenty of fluids to support recovery.
EAT NUTRITIOUS FOODS
Fuel your body with healthy foods.
FOLLOW DOCTOR'S ADVICE
Take prescribed medications as directed.
MANAGE STRESS
Use relaxation techniques like breathing or yoga.
WHEN TO SEEK MEDICAL HELP
• Fatigue lasts more than 2–4 weeks
• Symptoms are getting worse
• Trouble breathing or chest pain
• High fever that doesn't go away
• Fatigue affects daily life
KEY TAKEAWAY
Infections can cause fatigue, but most people recover with rest, good nutrition, and proper care. If fatigue lasts long or is severe, talk to your doctor.

A Patient Example

A 52-year-old man had a viral illness three months ago.

The fever settled, but he continued to feel tired. He tried to return to his usual exercise routine, but each time he pushed himself, he felt worse the next day.

He became frustrated and confused.

His pattern suggests post-exertional fatigue.

Instead of pushing harder, he needs a slower, paced approach to recovery.

Understanding this prevents further setbacks.

Doctor's Pearl

Not all fatigue improves with effort.

Sometimes the body needs time, pacing, and patience.

Common Mistakes to Avoid

- Assuming you should "push through" after illness
- Ignoring worsening symptoms after activity
- Remaining completely inactive for long periods
- Expecting quick recovery after significant illness
- Self-diagnosing without proper evaluation
- Becoming discouraged by slow progress

Chapter Summary

Infections can lead to prolonged fatigue even after the main illness has resolved. Long COVID and chronic fatigue syndrome may involve persistent tiredness, brain fog, and worsening of symptoms after activity. Recovery often requires a balanced approach with gradual activity and proper rest rather than extremes. Understanding the pattern of fatigue is essential for safe and effective recovery.

Action Plan

- Observe how your body responds to activity
- Avoid sudden increases in physical or mental effort
- Balance activity with rest
- Keep a simple record of symptoms and triggers
- Seek medical evaluation if fatigue persists beyond expected recovery
- Discuss pacing strategies with your doctor if symptoms worsen after exertion

Looking Ahead

Infections are one cause of fatigue, but medicines and substances can also quietly drain your energy.

In the next chapter, we will explore how prescription medicines, over-the-counter drugs, alcohol, caffeine, and supplements may contribute to tiredness, often in ways people do not recognize.

CHAPTER 13: Medicines, Alcohol, and Hidden Causes

When the Treatment Becomes Part of the Problem

Medicines can help us live longer and better.

They control blood pressure, reduce pain, improve mood, treat infections, help sleep, lower cholesterol, and protect the heart. Many medicines are necessary and should not be stopped without medical advice.

But sometimes, medicines can quietly contribute to tiredness.

The effect may be obvious, but often it is subtle. A patient starts a new medicine, increases a dose, adds an over-the-counter product, or begins taking several medicines together. Weeks later, they feel tired and do not connect the two.

That is why every evaluation of fatigue should include one simple step:

Review everything you take.

Prescription Medicines That May Cause Fatigue

Many prescription medicines can cause tiredness in some people.

Blood pressure medicines may lower blood pressure or heart rate enough to cause fatigue, lightheadedness, or reduced stamina.

Pain medicines, especially stronger ones, can cause drowsiness, mental slowing, constipation, and poor sleep quality.

Medicines for anxiety or sleep may relax the body at night but leave a person feeling dull the next morning.

Some antidepressants may initially cause tiredness or sleep changes, although they may be very helpful when properly used.

This does not mean these medicines are bad. It means they must be used thoughtfully.

Over-the-Counter Medicines Are Still Medicines

Many people forget to mention non-prescription medicines.

Allergy pills, cold medicines, sleep aids, motion sickness medicines, and some pain relievers can all affect energy, alertness, and balance.

This is especially important in older adults, who may be more sensitive to sedating effects.

A medicine bought without a prescription can still cause real side effects.

Polypharmacy: When Small Effects Add Up

Polypharmacy means taking several medicines at the same time.

Sometimes this is necessary. Many people live with several chronic conditions and need multiple treatments.

But the more medicines a person takes, the greater the chance of side effects, drug interactions, dizziness, sleepiness, confusion, poor appetite, or fatigue.

One medicine may cause mild tiredness. Another may cause mild dizziness. A third may disturb sleep. Together, they can create a major problem.

This is why a medication review with your doctor or pharmacist can be very valuable.

Alcohol and Sleep Quality

Alcohol can be a hidden cause of fatigue.

Many people use alcohol to relax or fall asleep. It may make you sleepy at first, but it often disturbs sleep later in the night. Sleep becomes lighter, more fragmented, and less restorative.

Alcohol can also interact with medicines, especially sleep medicines, anxiety medicines, pain medicines, and some antidepressants.

The person may not feel intoxicated, but the next day they may feel tired, foggy, and slow.

Caffeine: Helpful, but Not a Cure

Caffeine can improve alertness for a short time.

But caffeine is not treatment for fatigue. It is a temporary stimulant.

When used too late in the day, it can interfere with sleep. Then poor sleep leads to morning tiredness, and morning tiredness leads to more caffeine.

This cycle is common.

Coffee or tea in moderation is fine for many people. But when caffeine becomes your main energy strategy, it is time to look deeper.

Supplements and Energy Products

Many products promise more energy.

Some contain vitamins. Others contain herbs, stimulants, powders, or mixtures with long ingredient lists. A few may help in specific situations, but many are not well proven.

Some can interact with prescription medicines. Some may affect blood pressure, heart rhythm, sleep, liver function, or bleeding risk. Some may simply waste money and delay proper diagnosis.

Natural does not always mean safe.

If you take supplements, tell your doctor. This information matters.

MEDICINES, ALCOHOL AND OTHER CAUSES OF FATIGUE

MANY EVERYDAY FACTORS CAN DRAIN YOUR ENERGY AND CAUSE ONGOING FATIGUE.

MEDICINES THAT CAN CAUSE FATIGUE

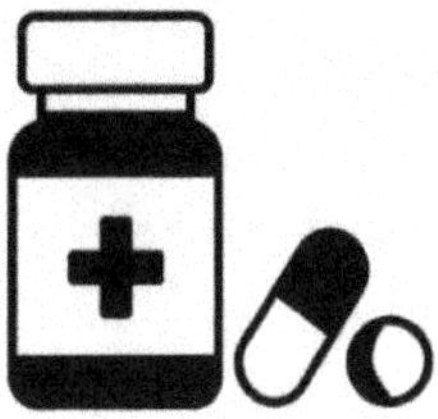

- PAIN RELIEVERS
- ANTIDEPRESSANTS
- ANTIHISTAMINES
- BLOOD PRESSURE MEDICINES
- MUSCLE RELAXANTS
- STEROIDS
- CHEMOTHERAPY DRUGS

ALWAYS TALK TO YOUR DOCTOR IF YOU FEEL UNUSUALLY TIRED.

ALCOHOL AND FATIGUE

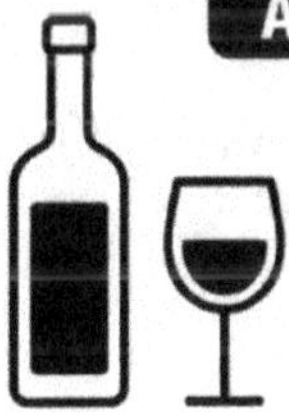

- DISTURBS SLEEP
- DEHYDRATES THE BODY
- AFFECTS NUTRIENT ABSORPTION
- OVERUSE CAN LEAD TO CHRONIC FATIGUE

DRINK IN MODERATION. TOO MUCH LEADS TO FATIGUE.

OTHER CAUSES OF FATIGUE

- POOR DIET
- DEHYDRATION
- LACK OF PHYSICAL ACTIVITY
- STRESS AND WORRY
- POOR SLEEP HABITS

Timing Can Make a Difference

Sometimes the issue is not the medicine itself, but timing.

A medicine that causes drowsiness may be better taken in the evening if your doctor agrees. A medicine that increases urination may disturb sleep if taken too late. A stimulant taken late may prevent sleep.

Small timing changes can sometimes improve energy significantly.

But do not change medication timing without asking your clinician, especially for heart, blood pressure, diabetes, seizure, psychiatric, or steroid medicines.

A Patient Example

A 72-year-old man complains of morning tiredness and fogginess.

He takes a sleep aid at night, an allergy pill, a pain medicine, and a muscle relaxer. He also drinks alcohol in the evening because it helps him unwind.

His blood tests are normal.

But his fatigue is not mysterious. Several substances may be affecting his sleep, alertness, and balance.

The answer is not to stop everything suddenly. The answer is a careful medication review and a safer plan.

Doctor's Pearl

Always ask, "Could something I am taking be taking my energy away?"

This includes prescriptions, over-the-counter medicines, vitamins, supplements, alcohol, caffeine, and recreational substances.

Common Mistakes to Avoid

- Stopping prescribed medicines suddenly
- Assuming over-the-counter medicines are harmless
- Forgetting to mention supplements
- Mixing alcohol with sedating medicines
- Using caffeine as the main treatment for fatigue
- Ignoring fatigue that began after a new medicine or dose change
- Taking multiple "energy" products without medical guidance

Chapter Summary

Medicines, alcohol, caffeine, supplements, and over-the-counter products can all contribute to tiredness. Sometimes thc effect is direct. Sometimes it comes from poor sleep, drug interactions, low blood pressure, sedation, or medication timing. A complete review of everything you take is an essential part of evaluating persistent fatigue.

Action Plan

- Make a complete list of all prescription medicines
- Add over-the-counter medicines, vitamins, supplements, sleep aids, and herbal products

- Include alcohol, caffeine, cannabis, or other substances if used
- Write down the dose and time you take each item
- Notice whether fatigue began after a new medicine or dose change
- Review the list with your doctor or pharmacist
- Do not stop important medicines without medical advice

Looking Ahead

Now that we have reviewed the major causes of tiredness, the next step is understanding how doctors put the clues together.

In the next chapter, we will discuss how constant tiredness is evaluated, why your story matters, which tests may be useful, and why thoughtful diagnosis is better than random testing.

CHAPTER 14: How Doctors Evaluate Constant Tiredness

The Right Diagnosis Begins with the Right Story

When a patient says, "Doctor, I am tired all the time," the best next step is not to order every possible test.

The best next step is to listen carefully.

Fatigue is a broad symptom. It may come from sleep problems, stress, anemia, thyroid disease, diabetes, depression, medications, chronic illness, infection, inflammation, poor nutrition, or many other causes. If testing is done without direction, it may create confusion rather than clarity.

Good medical evaluation follows a thoughtful path:

Listen carefully.
Examine properly.
Test wisely.
Follow up if needed.

This approach is simple, but powerful.

Why Your Story Matters So Much

Your story often gives the first and most important clue.

Your doctor may ask:

When did the tiredness begin?
Did it start suddenly or slowly?

Is it getting better, worse, or staying the same?
Do you feel sleepy, weak, breathless, foggy, or emotionally drained?
Does rest help?
Does activity make it worse?
How is your sleep?
Has your weight changed?
Do you have fever, pain, bleeding, or shortness of breath?
What medicines and supplements do you take?

These questions are not routine small talk. They guide the entire evaluation.

A clear story can prevent unnecessary testing and help identify the real problem sooner.

Looking for Patterns

Fatigue rarely travels alone.

It usually comes with clues.

Fatigue with loud snoring and daytime sleepiness may point toward sleep apnea.
Fatigue with heavy bleeding may suggest anemia.
Fatigue with weight gain, cold intolerance, and constipation may suggest thyroid disease.
Fatigue with thirst and frequent urination may suggest diabetes.
Fatigue with sadness, poor sleep, and loss of interest may suggest depression.
Fatigue after infection with worsening after activity may suggest post-illness fatigue.

Patterns matter.

One symptom may be vague. A group of symptoms becomes a direction.

The Physical Examination

A careful examination can reveal clues that the patient may not notice.

Your doctor may check:

Blood pressure and pulse
Weight changes
Oxygen level
Heart and lung findings
Thyroid gland
Skin and eyes
Abdomen
Leg swelling
Muscle strength
Neurological signs

The examination helps connect your symptoms with your body's findings.

Sometimes the examination is normal. That is still useful. It helps narrow the possibilities.

Common Blood Tests

Blood tests are often helpful, but they should be chosen thoughtfully.

Common initial tests may include:

Complete blood count to look for anemia or infection
Thyroid testing

Blood sugar or A1c
Kidney function
Liver function
Electrolytes
Iron studies when indicated
Vitamin B12 or vitamin D when appropriate
Urine testing in selected cases

These tests can detect many treatable causes of fatigue.

But no blood test explains every case of tiredness.

When Special Testing Is Needed

Sometimes the story points beyond basic blood tests.

If sleep apnea is suspected, a sleep study may be needed.

If fatigue comes with chest discomfort, palpitations, leg swelling, or shortness of breath, heart evaluation may be appropriate.

If lung disease is suspected, breathing tests or imaging may be needed.

If autoimmune disease is possible, more specific blood tests or specialist evaluation may be necessary.

The key is targeted testing.

Tests should answer a question, not replace thinking.

When Tests Are Normal

Many patients feel discouraged when tests come back normal.

They may think, "Then why do I feel so bad?"

Normal tests are useful. They rule out many important conditions. But they do not mean the fatigue is imaginary.

Fatigue may still come from sleep disorders, stress, depression, anxiety, medication effects, deconditioning, poor sleep rhythm, Long COVID, chronic fatigue syndrome, or other causes that may not appear on routine blood work.

If symptoms continue, follow-up matters.

A normal first evaluation is not always the end of the journey.

Why Follow-Up Is Important

Fatigue may change over time.

New symptoms may appear. Patterns may become clearer. A treatment trial may help or fail. A medicine adjustment may make a difference. A sleep diary may reveal a hidden problem.

This is why follow-up is essential.

Do not disappear from care if you still feel unwell. Return with more information. Bring your symptom diary. Bring your medication list. Tell your doctor what has changed.

Diagnosis is sometimes a process, not a single visit.

A Patient Example

A 58-year-old woman comes to the office because she is tired every day.

Her blood tests are normal. At first, she feels disappointed. But her story shows that she wakes unrefreshed, snores loudly, and feels sleepy during the day. Her doctor recommends evaluation for sleep apnea.

Another patient has fatigue, dizziness, and shortness of breath with stairs. Her blood count shows anemia.

A third patient has fatigue, low mood, poor sleep, and loss of interest. Depression becomes an important part of the evaluation.

Same complaint. Different pathways.

This is why the story matters.

Doctor's Pearl

The best diagnosis often begins before the first test is ordered.

Your history is not less important than your lab work. In many cases, it is more important.

Common Mistakes to Avoid

Do not demand every possible test without a clear reason.

Do not assume normal tests mean nothing is wrong.

Do not hide symptoms such as snoring, mood changes, alcohol use, bleeding, or medication side effects.

Do not stop follow-up if tiredness continues.

Do not rely only on internet searches.

Do not forget to bring a complete medication and supplement list.

Chapter Summary

Evaluating constant tiredness requires a careful and organized approach. The patient's story, symptom pattern, physical examination, and targeted testing all work together. Blood tests are useful, but they do not explain every case. When tests are normal but symptoms continue, follow-up is important. The goal is not random testing, but thoughtful diagnosis.

Action Plan

- Write down when your fatigue began
- Note whether it is improving, worsening, or staying the same
- Track sleep, meals, activity, stress, caffeine, alcohol, and symptoms
- Bring a complete list of medicines and supplements
- Tell your doctor about snoring, sleepiness, bleeding, weight change, mood symptoms, pain, breathlessness, or fever
- Ask which tests are appropriate and why
- Follow up if symptoms persist or change

Looking Ahead

Once the cause of tiredness is being explored, treatment can begin in a practical and safe way.

In the next chapter, we will discuss lifestyle treatment, the foundation of recovery, including sleep, food, hydration, movement, stress control, and daily rhythm.

CHAPTER 15: Lifestyle Treatment: The Foundation of Recovery

The First Treatment Is Often Not a Pill

When people feel tired all the time, they often ask, "What can I take to feel better?"

It is a natural question.

Sometimes medicine is necessary. If fatigue is caused by anemia, thyroid disease, diabetes, sleep apnea, depression, heart disease, kidney disease, or another medical condition, proper treatment is important.

But even when medicine is needed, the foundation of recovery usually begins with daily habits.

Sleep. Food. Water. Movement. Stress control. Routine.

These may sound simple, but they are not small. They are the basic systems that support energy every day. When they are weak, energy becomes weak. When they improve, the body often begins to feel stronger.

Sleep: The First Pillar of Energy

Sleep is where recovery begins.

A tired body needs restorative sleep, not just more time in bed. A regular sleep pattern helps the brain, hormones, muscles, and immune system function better.

Start with one simple rule: keep a consistent wake-up time.

This helps reset the body's internal clock. From there, create a calm evening routine. Reduce screens before bed. Avoid heavy meals late at night. Limit caffeine after lunch. Avoid alcohol as a sleep aid. Keep the bedroom dark, quiet, and comfortable.

If you snore loudly, wake up gasping, or feel sleepy during the day, do not treat this only as poor sleep. Ask your doctor whether sleep apnea should be considered.

Food: Steady Fuel for a Steady Body

Food should support energy, not create energy crashes.

Many tired people skip meals, eat irregularly, rely on coffee, or grab sweets for quick relief. This may help briefly, but the body soon feels drained again.

A better approach is simple:

Eat regular meals.
Include protein.
Choose fruits and vegetables.
Use whole grains when possible.
Limit heavy sugar intake.
Avoid using caffeine as a meal replacement.

You do not need a perfect diet. You need a steady, nourishing one.

Hydration: A Small Habit with Big Value

Water is often forgotten.

Even mild dehydration can make a person feel tired, lightheaded, headachy, or mentally dull. Many people drink coffee or tea all day but very little water.

Try drinking water regularly through the day. Watch your urine color, thirst, dizziness, and headaches. If you have heart failure, kidney disease, or another condition requiring fluid restriction, follow your doctor's advice.

Hydration should be sensible, not excessive.

Movement: Begin Gently

When you are tired, exercise may feel impossible.

But complete inactivity often worsens fatigue over time. Muscles lose strength. Stamina drops. Simple tasks begin to feel harder.

The solution is not sudden intense exercise. The solution is gentle, gradual movement.

Begin where you are.

For some, that may be a ten-minute walk. For others, it may be stretching, chair exercises, or walking inside the house.

The goal is consistency.

If activity makes you much worse the next day, or if you have chest pain, severe shortness of breath, fainting, or post-exertional worsening, speak with your doctor before increasing activity.

LIFESTYLE TREATMENT FOR FATIGUE

SIMPLE DAILY HABITS THAT CAN IMPROVE YOUR ENERGY AND REDUCE FATIGUE.

1. GET QUALITY SLEEP

SLEEP 7–9 HOURS EVERY NIGHT.
KEEP A REGULAR SLEEP SCHEDULE.

2. EAT A BALANCED DIET

EAT NUTRITIOUS FOODS, INCLUDING FRUITS, VEGETABLES, WHOLE GRAINS, PROTEIN, AND HEALTHY FATS.
AVOID TOO MUCH SUGAR AND PROCESSED FOODS.

3. STAY HYDRATED

DRINK ENOUGH WATER THROUGHOUT THE DAY.
DEHYDRATION CAN CAUSE TIREDNESS.

4. EXERCISE REGULARLY

DO MODERATE EXERCISE MOST DAYS OF THE WEEK.
EVEN 30 MINUTES A DAY CAN BOOST ENERGY.

5. MANAGE STRESS

PRACTICE RELAXATION TECHNIQUES LIKE DEEP BREATHING, MEDITATION, OR YOGA.
REDUCING STRESS IMPROVES ENERGY.

6. GET NATURAL SUNLIGHT

SPEND TIME IN NATURAL SUNLIGHT EVERY DAY.
IT HELPS REGULATE MOOD AND ENERGY.

7. PLAN YOUR DAY

TAKE BREAKS, PRIORITIZE TASKS, AND AVOID OVEREXERTION.
PACE YOURSELF THROUGHOUT THE DAY.

8. AVOID SMOKING AND LIMIT ALCOHOL

THEY CAN INCREASE FATIGUE AND AFFECT SLEEP AND OVERALL HEALTH.

Stress Control: Giving the Body Permission to Recover

Stress keeps the body on alert.

If that alert state continues for too long, sleep worsens, muscles tighten, appetite changes, and energy drops. Stress control is not a luxury. It is part of medical recovery.

Simple steps can help:

Take short quiet breaks.
Practice slow breathing.
Spend time outdoors.
Write down worries before bed.
Talk to someone you trust.
Reduce unnecessary evening stimulation.
Ask for help when responsibilities are too heavy.

You may not be able to remove all stress, but you can give your body moments of recovery.

Daily Rhythm: The Body Likes Regularity

The body works best with rhythm.

Regular wake times, meals, movement, light exposure, work, rest, and bedtime help stabilize energy. Irregular days make the body work harder to adjust.

A simple rhythm may look like this:

Wake at a consistent time.
Get morning light.
Eat breakfast or an early balanced meal.

Move gently.
Drink water.
Limit late caffeine.
Begin winding down before bedtime.

These steps are ordinary, but when repeated, they become powerful.

Do Not Try to Fix Everything at Once

One common mistake is trying to change too much too quickly.

A tired person may decide to start a strict diet, exercise daily, stop caffeine completely, sleep earlier, take supplements, and reorganize life all in one week.

That usually fails.

Choose one or two changes first. Let them become stable. Then add more.

Recovery is built step by step.

A Patient Example

A 61-year-old woman feels tired every day. Her basic tests are reassuring, but her routine is irregular. She sleeps late, wakes at different times, drinks coffee in the afternoon, skips breakfast, and has stopped walking.

Her plan is simple.

She sets a regular wake-up time. She stops caffeine after lunch. She adds a protein-containing breakfast. She drinks water regularly. She walks for ten minutes after dinner.

After three weeks, she is not completely cured, but she feels clearer and more in control.

This is how many recoveries begin, not with a dramatic change, but with steady correction of daily habits.

Doctor's Pearl

Lifestyle treatment is not "minor treatment."

It is the foundation that helps the body respond to everything else.

Common Mistakes to Avoid

- Trying to change everything at once
- Using caffeine instead of sleep
- Skipping meals and expecting steady energy
- Starting intense exercise too quickly
- Ignoring sleep apnea symptoms
- Drinking alcohol to fall asleep
- Giving up because improvement is gradual

Chapter Summary

Lifestyle treatment is the foundation of fatigue recovery. Better sleep, steady nutrition, hydration, gentle movement, stress control, and daily rhythm can improve energy and support medical treatment. These steps do not replace medical care when disease is present, but they help almost every person build a healthier energy system.

Action Plan

- Keep a consistent wake-up time
- Create a calm evening routine
- Avoid caffeine late in the day
- Eat regular meals with protein
- Drink water regularly
- Begin gentle movement if safe
- Take short recovery breaks during the day
- Build one habit at a time
- Seek medical advice if fatigue persists, worsens, or comes with warning signs

Looking Ahead

Lifestyle changes are powerful, but sometimes they are not enough.

In the next chapter, we will discuss medical treatment, including how doctors treat anemia, thyroid disease, diabetes, sleep apnea, depression, chronic illness, and medication-related fatigue by targeting the real cause.

CHAPTER 16: Medical Treatment: Treating the Real Cause

There Is No Single Pill for Tiredness

Many patients ask a very reasonable question:

“Doctor, what can I take to get my energy back?”

I understand that question. When a person is tired every day, they want relief. They want something that works quickly. They want their normal life back.

But constant tiredness does not have one universal treatment.

Tiredness is not one disease. It is a signal. The correct treatment depends on what is causing that signal.

If the cause is anemia, the treatment is different.
If the cause is sleep apnea, the treatment is different.
If the cause is depression, thyroid disease, diabetes, medication side effects, heart disease, kidney disease, or chronic inflammation, the treatment is different again.

The best medical care does not simply cover fatigue. It asks, “What is taking your energy away?”

Treating Anemia and Deficiencies

When fatigue is caused by anemia or nutritional deficiency, treatment must be specific.

Iron deficiency requires iron replacement, but it also requires finding out why iron is low. In a young woman, heavy menstrual bleeding may be the reason. In an older adult, hidden blood loss from the stomach or intestine may need evaluation.

Vitamin B12 deficiency may require oral supplements or injections, depending on the cause and severity. This is important because B12 affects not only energy, but also nerves, memory, balance, and blood formation.

Vitamin D deficiency may be treated when levels are low, especially when muscle weakness, bone health, or other risk factors are present.

The goal is not to take vitamins randomly. The goal is to correct what is truly missing.

Treating Thyroid and Hormonal Problems

If the thyroid is underactive, replacing thyroid hormone can gradually improve energy, mental clarity, weight pattern, bowel function, and cold intolerance.

If the thyroid is overactive, treatment depends on the cause and may include medication, radioactive iodine, or other specialist-guided care.

Blood sugar problems require careful management. In diabetes, fatigue may improve when blood sugar becomes more stable, dehydration improves, sleep improves, and complications are addressed.

Hormone treatment should never be used casually as an "energy booster." These treatments are powerful and should be based on proper diagnosis, appropriate testing, and follow-up.

Treating Sleep Disorders

If sleep apnea is the cause, treatment can make a major difference.

Positive airway pressure therapy, oral appliances, weight management when appropriate, positional changes, or other treatments may be used depending on the type and severity of sleep apnea.

For insomnia, treatment may include improving sleep habits, treating pain or anxiety, cognitive behavioral therapy for insomnia, and sometimes carefully selected medications.

The goal is not simply to sedate the patient. The goal is to restore healthy sleep.

Good sleep is one of the strongest medicines for fatigue.

Treating Depression, Anxiety, and Burnout

When fatigue is connected with depression or anxiety, treatment can be life-changing.

Treatment may include counseling, cognitive behavioral therapy, stress management, better sleep, exercise when appropriate, social support, and medication when needed.

This is not "just emotional."

The brain is part of the body. When mood improves, sleep, motivation, appetite, concentration, and physical energy often improve as well.

Burnout may require a different kind of treatment: boundaries, rest, workload adjustment, family support, time away from constant pressure, and sometimes professional counseling.

Managing Chronic Diseases

When tiredness comes from heart disease, lung disease, kidney disease, liver disease, autoimmune disease, or other chronic illness, the goal is to treat and control that condition as well as possible.

For some diseases, fatigue improves greatly when the condition is treated. For others, the goal may be better management rather than complete cure.

This may include medicines, rehabilitation, oxygen therapy when needed, better nutrition, physical therapy, disease monitoring, or specialist care.

The key is realistic progress.

Improvement may come slowly, but even partial improvement can greatly improve daily life.

Adjusting Medicines That Cause Fatigue

Sometimes the best treatment is not adding a new medicine.

Sometimes it is adjusting an old one.

A medication may be causing drowsiness, low blood pressure, poor sleep, dizziness, or mental fog. Your doctor may adjust the dose, change the timing, switch to another medicine, or reduce unnecessary medications.

This must be done carefully.

Do not stop blood pressure medicines, heart medicines, seizure medicines, antidepressants, steroids, sleep medicines, or pain medicines suddenly without medical guidance.

Safe adjustment is a medical decision.

When Specialist Care Is Needed

Sometimes fatigue requires a specialist.

A cardiologist may be needed for heart symptoms.
A pulmonologist may be needed for lung disease or sleep apnea.
An endocrinologist may be needed for difficult thyroid, diabetes, or hormonal problems.
A hematologist may be needed for unexplained anemia.
A rheumatologist may be needed for autoimmune disease.
A neurologist may be needed for true weakness or neurological symptoms.
A mental health professional may be needed for depression, anxiety, trauma, or burnout.

Referral does not always mean something frightening. It means the problem needs more focused expertise.

Good care is teamwork.

MEDICAL TREATMENT FOR FATIGUE

DOCTOR-DIRECTED TREATMENTS TO FIND THE CAUSE AND IMPROVE YOUR ENERGY.

1. TREAT THE UNDERLYING CAUSE

DOCTORS IDENTIFY AND TREAT CONDITIONS LIKE ANEMIA, THYROID DISORDERS, DIABETES, INFECTIONS, HORMONAL IMBALANCES, OR CHRONIC DISEASES.

2. MEDICATIONS

SPECIFIC MEDICINES MAY BE PRESCRIBED TO TREAT THE UNDERLYING CONDITION CAUSING FATIGUE, SUCH AS THYROID MEDICATION OR IRON SUPPLEMENTS.

3. VITAMIN AND MINERAL SUPPLEMENTS

SUPPLEMENTS LIKE IRON, VITAMIN B12, VITAMIN D, OR MAGNESIUM MAY BE PRESCRIBED IF DEFICIENCIES ARE FOUND.

4. TREAT SLEEP DISORDERS

CONDITIONS LIKE SLEEP APNEA OR INSOMNIA ARE TREATED WITH MEDICATIONS OR THERAPIES TO IMPROVE SLEEP QUALITY AND REDUCE FATIGUE.

5. MANAGE MENTAL HEALTH CONDITIONS

ANTIDEPRESSANTS, ANXIETY MEDICATIONS, OR COUNSELING CAN HELP TREAT DEPRESSION, ANXIETY, AND STRESS THAT MAY CAUSE FATIGUE.

6. MANAGE CHRONIC PAIN OR ILLNESS

MEDICATIONS, PHYSIOTHERAPY, OR OTHER THERAPIES CAN HELP MANAGE CHRONIC PAIN, ARTHRITIS, OR AUTOIMMUNE DISEASES THAT LEAD TO FATIGUE.

7. IV FLUIDS OR NUTRITION THERAPY

IN SOME CASES, IV FLUIDS, B12 INJECTIONS, OR NUTRITION THERAPY MAY BE USED TO IMPROVE ENERGY LEVELS.

8. REGULAR FOLLOW-UP

REGULAR CHECK-UPS HELP MONITOR PROGRESS, ADJUST TREATMENTS, AND ENSURE LONG-TERM IMPROVEMENT.

ALWAYS FOLLOW YOUR DOCTOR'S ADVICE AND COMPLETE THE FULL COURSE OF TREATMENT FOR BEST RESULTS.

Realistic Expectations

Medical treatment takes time.

Iron stores may take weeks or months to rebuild. Thyroid symptoms may improve gradually after treatment begins. Sleep apnea treatment may help quickly for some people, but others need time to adjust. Depression and anxiety treatment also take time.

Do not judge treatment too early.

At the same time, do not ignore lack of progress. If fatigue does not improve, follow up. The diagnosis may need to be reconsidered. Another cause may be present. The treatment plan may need adjustment.

Recovery is often a process.

A Patient Example

A 56-year-old man feels tired every day.

He assumes he needs vitamins. But evaluation shows untreated sleep apnea, high blood sugar, and a blood pressure medicine that may be contributing to low energy.

His treatment is not one pill.

He begins sleep apnea treatment, improves blood sugar control, reviews medicines with his doctor, and gradually increases activity.

After several months, his energy is much better.

This is common in real life. Fatigue often improves when several energy drains are addressed together.

Doctor's Pearl

Do not ask only, "What can I take for energy?"

Ask, "What is taking my energy away, and how can we treat it safely?"

Common Mistakes to Avoid

- Expecting one pill to fix all fatigue
- Taking supplements without knowing the cause
- Stopping prescribed medicines suddenly
- Ignoring follow-up appointments
- Comparing your recovery with someone else's
- Giving up too soon when treatment takes time
- Forgetting that several causes may exist together

Chapter Summary

Medical treatment for tiredness depends on the cause. Anemia, vitamin deficiencies, thyroid disease, diabetes, sleep disorders, depression, anxiety, chronic disease, and medication side effects all require different approaches. The best treatment is specific, evidence-based, safe, and guided by proper evaluation. Many people improve when the real cause is found and treated carefully.

Action Plan

- Ask your doctor what specific cause is being treated
- Understand what improvement should look like and how long it may take

- Take medicines as directed
- Report side effects promptly
- Do not stop medicines suddenly without guidance
- Keep follow-up appointments
- Continue lifestyle foundations while medical treatment is underway
- Ask whether specialist care is needed if fatigue persists

Looking Ahead

Medical treatment is important, but medicine continues to evolve.

In the next chapter, we will look at new and emerging approaches, including wearable devices, sleep technology, Long COVID research, chronic fatigue research, personalized care, and how to separate real progress from false promises.

CHAPTER 17: New and Emerging Approaches

Hope with Clear Thinking

When tiredness lasts for a long time, people naturally look for new answers.

They may read about wearable devices, sleep apps, genetic testing, special supplements, "energy boosters," Long COVID clinics, advanced blood tests, and personalized medicine.

Some of these tools can be useful. Some are promising. Some are still being studied. And some are not proven at all.

This chapter is about balance.

We should welcome progress, but we should also be careful. A tired person needs honest guidance, not false hope.

Wearable Devices and Health Tracking

Many people now use smartwatches, rings, and phone apps to track sleep, heart rate, oxygen levels, steps, and daily activity.

These tools can be helpful when used wisely.

They may show that your sleep is irregular, your activity level has dropped, your heart rate rises quickly, or your nighttime oxygen level may need attention. This information can start a useful conversation with your doctor.

But wearable devices do not replace medical evaluation.

They can show patterns. They cannot fully diagnose the cause of fatigue.

Sleep Technology

Home sleep technology is improving.

Some devices can give clues about snoring, oxygen drops, restlessness, and sleep timing. These tools may help you notice problems you would otherwise miss.

But if sleep apnea or another sleep disorder is suspected, proper medical testing may still be needed.

A sleep app can suggest that sleep is poor. A medical evaluation helps explain why.

Long COVID Research

Long COVID has brought new attention to persistent fatigue after infection.

Many people with Long COVID describe tiredness, brain fog, poor sleep, shortness of breath, palpitations, dizziness, and worsening symptoms after activity.

Research is continuing, and understanding is improving. But there is still no single cure for Long COVID fatigue.

Treatment usually focuses on careful evaluation, pacing of activity, sleep support, symptom management, rehabilitation when appropriate, and treatment of associated problems.

This is an area where medicine is still learning.

Chronic Fatigue Syndrome Research

Chronic fatigue syndrome, also called ME/CFS, remains a complex and often misunderstood condition.

One of its key features is worsening of symptoms after physical or mental effort. This is why simply telling every tired person to exercise harder is not always correct.

Research continues into immune changes, nervous system function, metabolism, circulation, sleep, and inflammation.

There is still much to learn, but recognition of this condition has improved. That matters, because patients need understanding as well as treatment.

Personalized Medicine

Personalized medicine means tailoring care to the individual.

In fatigue, this is especially important.

One person may need treatment for anemia. Another may need sleep apnea treatment. Another may need depression care. Another may need medication adjustment. Another may need pacing after Long COVID.

There is no single fatigue pathway for everyone.

The future of medicine may bring better ways to identify fatigue subtypes and match patients with more precise treatment. But even today, good care begins with personalized listening.

Supplements and Energy Products

Many products are marketed for energy.

Some contain vitamins. Some contain herbs. Some contain stimulants. Some claim to support mitochondria, detoxification, adrenal health, or immune balance.

Be careful.

Some products may help in selected situations, especially when a true deficiency exists. But many are not well proven. Some may interact with medications or cause side effects. Others may simply delay proper diagnosis.

A testimonial is not the same as scientific evidence.

Natural does not always mean safe.

Advanced Testing: Useful or Unnecessary?

Some patients are offered large panels of advanced tests.

In certain situations, specialized testing is appropriate. But more testing is not always better.

Unnecessary tests may create anxiety, confusion, and expense. Results may be difficult to interpret. Some abnormalities may not be related to fatigue at all.

Testing should answer a meaningful clinical question.

The best approach is not “test everything.” The best approach is “test wisely.”

A Patient Example

A 58-year-old woman uses a smartwatch and notices poor sleep scores almost every night. She also sees drops in oxygen during sleep.

Instead of buying supplements, she brings this information to her doctor. Further evaluation suggests sleep apnea, and treatment improves her energy.

In this case, technology helped because it guided proper medical care.

Another patient spends hundreds of dollars on energy supplements without improvement. Later, basic testing shows iron deficiency anemia.

The lesson is clear: new tools are useful only when they lead to better understanding.

Doctor’s Pearl

Technology can collect data, but wisdom must interpret it.

The best care combines modern tools with careful listening, sound medical judgment, and common sense.

Common Mistakes to Avoid

- Treating wearable data as a final diagnosis
- Spending large amounts on unproven energy treatments
- Ignoring basic causes while chasing rare explanations
- Taking supplements without medical guidance
- Believing every health claim online
- Assuming newer always means better
- Losing hope because research is still evolving

Chapter Summary

New and emerging approaches may improve how we understand fatigue. Wearables, sleep technology, Long COVID research, chronic fatigue syndrome research, personalized medicine, and advanced testing all have potential value. But these tools must be used carefully. The best approach is hopeful but realistic, open to progress but grounded in reliable medical care.

Action Plan

- Use wearable devices to observe patterns, not to diagnose yourself
- Share useful data with your doctor
- Be cautious with expensive supplements or fatigue programs
- Ask whether a test will truly change management
- Follow reliable medical guidance, not marketing claims

- Continue the basics: sleep, nutrition, hydration, movement, stress control, and medical follow-up
- Stay hopeful, but demand evidence

Looking Ahead

We have now reviewed the major causes, evaluation, treatment, and future directions of fatigue.

In the next chapter, we will bring everything together into a simple, practical plan that helps you move from confusion to action, one steady step at a time.

CHAPTER 18: A Simple, Practical Plan to Regain Your Energy

From Understanding to Action

By now, you have learned that tiredness is not one simple problem.

It may come from sleep disruption, stress, poor nutrition, anemia, thyroid disease, diabetes, chronic illness, infection, medications, inactivity, or several factors working together.

This can feel overwhelming.

But the answer is not to do everything at once. The answer is to move forward in a clear, organized way.

A tired person needs a plan that is simple enough to follow and strong enough to create progress.

Step 1: Observe Before You Change Everything

Before making major changes, spend a few days observing your pattern.

Ask yourself:

When did my tiredness begin?
Is it getting better, worse, or staying the same?
Do I feel sleepy, weak, breathless, foggy, or emotionally drained?

Do I wake refreshed or tired?
Does activity help or make things worse?
What medicines, supplements, caffeine, or alcohol am I using?
What has changed in my life recently?

Write the answers down.

Do not depend on memory alone. When you are tired, days blur together. A short written record can reveal patterns that the mind misses.

Step 2: Check for Warning Signs

Before starting a home plan, make sure there are no red flags.

Seek medical attention promptly if fatigue is associated with chest pain, severe shortness of breath, fainting, black stools, bleeding, unexplained weight loss, fever, night sweats, confusion, new neurological symptoms, or severe weakness.

These symptoms do not always mean something dangerous, but they should not be ignored.

Safety comes first.

Step 3: Strengthen the Foundation

Once urgent concerns are ruled out, begin with the basics.

These are the foundations of energy:

Sleep
Food
Water
Movement
Stress control
Daily rhythm

Choose one or two areas to improve first. Trying to change everything at once usually leads to frustration.

Start small, but start.

Step 4: Reset Your Sleep Routine

Sleep is the first place to begin for many people.

Set a regular wake-up time. Reduce caffeine after lunch. Avoid alcohol as a sleep aid. Create a quiet evening routine. Keep the bedroom dark, calm, and comfortable.

If you snore loudly, wake up gasping, feel sleepy during the day, or wake unrefreshed despite enough time in bed, ask your doctor whether a sleep disorder should be evaluated.

Do not assume poor sleep is just part of aging.

Step 5: Feed the Body Steadily

Energy needs steady fuel.

Eat regular meals. Include protein when possible. Add fruits, vegetables, and whole grains. Drink water through the day. Avoid using coffee as a substitute for food.

If you feel tired after large sugary meals, or if you crash in the afternoon, your meal pattern may need adjustment.

The goal is not a perfect diet. The goal is steadier energy.

Step 6: Move Gently and Consistently

Movement helps the body rebuild stamina.

If it is safe for you, begin with gentle activity. A short walk, light stretching, or simple chair exercises may be enough at first.

Do not start with intensity. Start with consistency.

If activity causes symptoms to worsen the next day or for several days, slow down and discuss this with your doctor. Some conditions require pacing rather than pushing.

Step 7: Review Stress and Emotional Load

Many people underestimate how much emotional strain drains the body.

Ask yourself:

Am I carrying too much?
Am I sleeping poorly because of worry?
Am I burned out?
Am I sad, anxious, or overwhelmed?
Do I need help?

Stress recovery may include quiet breaks, counseling, better boundaries, social support, journaling, time outdoors, or medical care when anxiety or depression is present.

Rest is not laziness. Rest is repair.

Step 8: Review Medicines and Supplements

Make a complete list of everything you take.

Include prescriptions, over-the-counter medicines, vitamins, herbal products, sleep aids, pain relievers, allergy medicines, alcohol, caffeine, and cannabis if used.

Look for changes.

Did fatigue begin after a new medicine?
Did it worsen after a dose change?
Are you taking several sedating products?

Review this list with your doctor or pharmacist. Do not stop important medicines on your own.

Step 9: Decide When Medical Evaluation Is Needed

A home plan is helpful, but it has limits.

You should seek medical evaluation if fatigue lasts several weeks, is worsening, affects daily function, or remains unexplained despite improving sleep, nutrition, hydration, activity, and routine.

Your doctor may consider blood tests, urine tests, sleep evaluation, heart or lung testing, medication review, or specialist referral based on your symptoms.

The purpose is not to order everything. The purpose is to look wisely.

Step 10: Build Slowly and Stay Patient

Recovery from fatigue is often gradual.

Some people improve within a few weeks. Others need months. Some improve partly, then need further evaluation. That is normal.

Do not judge your progress by one bad day.

Look for trends.

Are you waking a little better?
Walking a little farther?
Thinking a little more clearly?
Using less caffeine?
Feeling more in control?

Small gains matter.

A Simple 30-Day Starting Plan

Week 1: Observe and record your pattern. Track sleep, meals, caffeine, alcohol, activity, stress, medicines, and symptoms.

Week 2: Improve sleep routine. Keep a consistent wake time, reduce late caffeine, and create a calmer evening.

Week 3: Improve food, hydration, and movement. Eat regular meals, drink water, and begin gentle activity if safe.

Week 4: Review progress. Identify what helped, what did not, and whether medical evaluation or follow-up is needed.

This plan is not a cure for every cause of fatigue. It is a practical way to regain direction.

A Patient Example

A 60-year-old woman feels tired every day.

In the first week, she tracks her routine and notices that she sleeps irregularly, drinks coffee late, skips meals, and rarely moves.

In the second week, she fixes her wake-up time and stops caffeine after lunch.

In the third week, she adds breakfast with protein, drinks more water, and walks ten minutes daily.

By the fourth week, her energy is somewhat better, but she still wakes unrefreshed and snores loudly.

Her plan helped, but it also revealed the next step. She needs to discuss possible sleep apnea with her doctor.

That is progress.

Doctor's Pearl

A good plan does not have to solve everything immediately.

It must help you move from confusion to direction.

Common Mistakes to Avoid

- Trying to change everything at once
- Ignoring warning signs
- Starting intense exercise too quickly
- Depending on caffeine or supplements as shortcuts
- Stopping medicines without medical advice
- Giving up because improvement is slow
- Failing to follow up when symptoms persist

Chapter Summary

Improving fatigue requires a practical, step-by-step approach. Start by observing your pattern and checking for warning signs. Strengthen the basics: sleep, food, hydration, movement, stress control, routine, and medication review. Seek medical evaluation when fatigue is persistent, worsening, unexplained, or affecting daily life. Recovery often comes gradually, but steady progress can restore confidence and control.

Action Plan

- Track your fatigue pattern for at least one week
- Check for warning signs
- Choose one or two daily habits to improve first
- Set a consistent wake-up time
- Eat regular meals and drink water
- Begin gentle movement if safe
- Review medicines and supplements with your doctor or pharmacist
- Seek medical care if fatigue persists or worsens
- Measure progress by trends, not by one difficult day

Looking Ahead

You now have a practical plan to begin moving forward.

In the next chapter, we will answer the most common questions people ask about tiredness, including whether fatigue is just aging, whether vitamins help, what tests may be needed, and when to worry.

CHAPTER 19: Frequently Asked Questions About Tiredness

Questions Patients Ask Every Day

When people feel tired all the time, they usually have many questions.

They may not need a long medical lecture. They need clear, practical answers.

Is this just aging?
Do I need tests?
Will vitamins help?
Should I rest or exercise?
Why am I tired even after sleeping?
When should I worry?

These are important questions because the answers can guide the next step.

Is Tiredness Just Part of Aging?

Some change in stamina can happen with age.

You may not recover as quickly after a very busy day. Sleep patterns may change. Muscle strength may decrease if activity declines.

But constant tiredness should not be accepted as normal aging.

Many treatable problems become more common with age, including anemia, thyroid disease, diabetes, sleep apnea, depression, medication side effects, heart disease, kidney disease, and reduced physical conditioning.

Do not blame age too quickly.

Aging may change energy, but it should not take away your life.

Why Am I Tired Even After Sleeping?

This is one of the most common questions.

The answer is usually sleep quality.

You may spend enough hours in bed, but your sleep may be interrupted, shallow, poorly timed, or disturbed by sleep apnea, pain, stress, alcohol, medications, or restless legs.

If you wake up unrefreshed most mornings, your sleep deserves closer attention.

More hours in bed may not solve the problem if the sleep itself is not restorative.

Do I Need Blood Tests?

Not everyone needs extensive testing.

But if tiredness lasts for several weeks, is worsening, affects daily function, or has no clear explanation, basic testing is often useful.

Your doctor may check for anemia, thyroid disease, diabetes, kidney disease, liver problems, inflammation, vitamin deficiencies, or other conditions depending on your symptoms.

The goal is not to test everything.

The goal is to test wisely.

Can Vitamins Fix My Fatigue?

Vitamins help when there is a true deficiency.

Iron helps iron deficiency.
Vitamin B12 helps B12 deficiency.
Vitamin D helps when vitamin D is low.

But vitamins are not universal energy pills.

If your tiredness is caused by sleep apnea, depression, thyroid disease, medication side effects, heart disease, poor sleep, or stress, random vitamins may not help.

Supplements should support a diagnosis, not replace one.

Should I Exercise or Rest?

The answer depends on your pattern.

For many people, gentle movement improves energy over time. Walking, stretching, and light strengthening can rebuild stamina.

But some people feel worse after activity, especially if symptoms worsen the next day or last for several days. This pattern needs a more careful approach.

Do not jump from inactivity to heavy exercise.

Start gently. Increase slowly. Listen to your body. If exertion causes a delayed crash, discuss this with your doctor.

Why Are My Tests Normal If I Still Feel Bad?

This can be frustrating.

Normal tests are reassuring, but they do not explain every cause of fatigue.

Routine blood tests may not show poor sleep, sleep apnea, stress, depression, medication side effects, deconditioning, Long COVID, chronic fatigue syndrome, or burnout.

Normal tests do not mean your symptoms are fake.

They mean certain problems were not found. The next step is to look at the whole picture.

How Long Does Recovery Take?

Recovery depends on the cause.

Some people improve in a few weeks after correcting sleep, nutrition, hydration, or medication timing. Others need months, especially if fatigue is related to chronic illness, anemia, depression, Long COVID, or deconditioning.

Do not measure recovery by one day.

Look at the trend.

Are you doing a little more? Thinking more clearly? Sleeping better? Needing less caffeine? Recovering faster?

Small improvement is still improvement.

When Should I Worry?

You should seek medical care promptly if tiredness comes with:

- Chest pain or pressure
- Severe shortness of breath
- Fainting
- Black stools or bleeding
- Unexplained weight loss
- Fever or night sweats
- Confusion
- New neurological symptoms
- Severe weakness
- Thoughts of self-harm

You should also call your doctor if fatigue is persistent, worsening, unexplained, or interfering with daily life.

Can Fatigue Be Completely Cured?

Sometimes, yes.

If the cause is iron deficiency, thyroid disease, sleep apnea, medication side effects, poor sleep habits, or another correctable problem, energy may improve significantly.

In chronic conditions, the goal may be improvement rather than complete cure.

But improvement matters. Better energy, clearer thinking, safer function, and improved quality of life are meaningful goals.

Should I See a Specialist?

Not always.

Many cases of fatigue can be evaluated and managed by a primary care doctor.

A specialist may be needed if symptoms point toward a specific system, such as the heart, lungs, thyroid, blood, kidneys, immune system, nervous system, sleep disorder, or mental health condition.

Referral is not failure. It is focused care.

A Patient Example

A 57-year-old man says, "All my blood tests are normal, so I guess nothing is wrong."

But he wakes unrefreshed, snores loudly, drinks coffee late, naps in the afternoon, and feels sleepy while watching television.

His blood tests are normal, but his sleep may not be normal.

The next step is not to give up. The next step is to look more carefully.

Doctor's Pearl

A normal test result does not always mean a normal life.

If you still feel unwell, keep asking thoughtful questions and keep looking for the pattern.

Common Mistakes to Avoid

- Blaming all fatigue on age
- Taking vitamins without knowing whether you need them
- Ignoring sleep quality
- Assuming normal tests mean there is no problem
- Starting intense exercise too quickly
- Delaying care when warning signs are present
- Giving up when recovery is slow

Chapter Summary

Tiredness raises many common questions, and most have practical answers. Aging alone should not explain persistent fatigue. Sleep quality matters as much as sleep duration. Vitamins help only when a true deficiency exists. Testing should be guided by symptoms and examination. Exercise helps many people, but it must be gradual and appropriate. Normal tests do not rule out every cause. Recovery takes time, but improvement is often possible.

Action Plan

- Write down your top three questions before your doctor visit
- Track your sleep, energy, symptoms, medicines, caffeine, and activity

- Ask whether your fatigue pattern suggests sleep problems, anemia, thyroid disease, diabetes, medication effects, stress, or another cause
- Avoid random supplements unless a deficiency is identified
- Start movement gradually if safe
- Seek medical care if fatigue is persistent, worsening, unexplained, or associated with warning signs
- Focus on progress, not perfection

Looking Ahead

Even when we understand fatigue better, many myths still remain.

In the next chapter, we will separate common myths from facts, so you can avoid misleading advice and make better decisions about your health.

CHAPTER 20: Myths and Facts About Tiredness

Why Myths Can Delay Recovery

Tiredness is so common that people often explain it too quickly.

They say it is age.
They say it is stress.
They say they need more coffee.
They say vitamins will fix it.
They say normal blood tests mean nothing is wrong.

These explanations may sound harmless, but they can delay the right care.

A myth becomes dangerous when it stops a person from asking the right question.

The goal of this chapter is simple: separate what sounds true from what is actually true.

Myth 1: Tiredness Is Just Part of Aging

Aging can change stamina. Recovery may take longer. Sleep may become lighter. Muscle strength may decline if a person becomes inactive.

But constant tiredness should not be accepted as normal aging.

Fatigue in older adults may come from anemia, thyroid disease, diabetes, sleep apnea, depression, medication side effects, heart disease, kidney disease, poor nutrition, or reduced activity.

Fact: Aging may change energy, but it should not take away your life.

Myth 2: More Sleep Will Fix Everything

Sleep is essential, but more time in bed does not always mean better rest.

If sleep is interrupted by sleep apnea, insomnia, pain, stress, alcohol, restless legs, or medication effects, the body may not recover properly.

A person may sleep eight hours and still wake exhausted.

Fact: Sleep quality matters as much as sleep duration.

Myth 3: Coffee Is the Best Treatment for Fatigue

Coffee may improve alertness for a short time.

But caffeine does not treat the cause of fatigue. It can also disturb sleep, especially when taken later in the day.

This can create a cycle:

Tiredness leads to caffeine.
Caffeine worsens sleep.
Poor sleep causes more tiredness.

Fact: Caffeine may help briefly, but it is not a treatment plan.

Myth 4: Normal Blood Tests Mean Nothing Is Wrong

Normal tests are reassuring, but they do not explain everything.

Routine blood tests may miss sleep disorders, stress-related fatigue, medication effects, deconditioning, depression, anxiety, Long COVID, chronic fatigue syndrome, or burnout.

Normal results should not be ignored, but they should not end the conversation if symptoms continue.

Fact: Normal tests rule out some causes, not all causes.

Myth 5: Exercise Always Helps Fatigue

For many people, gentle movement improves energy over time.

But not everyone should push harder. Some people feel much worse after activity, especially those with post-exertional malaise, Long COVID, or chronic fatigue syndrome.

The right approach is gradual and individualized.

Fact: Movement helps many people, but the dose must fit the condition.

Myth 6: Vitamins Are Always Safe and Helpful

Vitamins help when the body truly needs them.

Iron helps iron deficiency. Vitamin B12 helps B12 deficiency. Vitamin D helps when vitamin D is low.

But random supplements are not magic energy pills. Some can cause side effects, interact with medicines, or delay diagnosis.

Fact: Supplements should be targeted, not guessed.

Myth 7: I Just Need to Push Through

Many people are proud of pushing through.

There are times in life when endurance is necessary. But constantly ignoring fatigue can make things worse. It may delay diagnosis, worsen burnout, increase mistakes, or deepen exhaustion.

Listening to your body is not weakness.

Fact: Rest, evaluation, and recovery are part of strength.

Myth 8: If It Were Serious, I Would Know

Not always.

Some conditions develop quietly. Fatigue may appear before obvious pain or dramatic symptoms. Heart disease, anemia, kidney disease, thyroid disease, sleep apnea, depression, and chronic illness may begin subtly.

The body does not always shout. Sometimes it whispers.

Fact: Persistent change in energy deserves attention.

Myth 9: All Fatigue Is Stress

Stress is a common cause of fatigue, but it is not the only cause.

Blaming everything on stress can be just as wrong as ignoring stress completely. A person may be stressed and still have anemia. They may be anxious and still have thyroid disease. They may be burned out and still have sleep apnea.

Fact: Stress matters, but the whole person must be evaluated.

Myth 10: One Treatment Should Fix Everything

Many people want one clear answer.

But fatigue is often caused by several factors together. Poor sleep, inactivity, stress, medication effects, and mild medical problems can combine.

Treatment may require several small corrections rather than one dramatic solution.

Fact: Energy often returns through a step-by-step plan.

A Patient Example

A 55-year-old woman believes her tiredness is just age.

She drinks more coffee, takes vitamins, and keeps pushing herself. Months later, she finally sees her doctor. Her tests show iron deficiency anemia from heavy menstrual bleeding.

Her fatigue was not age. It was a treatable problem.

Another patient believes vitamins will solve everything, but his main issue is loud snoring and unrefreshing sleep. His fatigue improves only after sleep apnea is diagnosed and treated.

Different myths. Same delay.

Doctor's Pearl

Quick explanations are not always correct explanations.

When fatigue persists, do not settle for a label. Look for the pattern.

Common Mistakes to Avoid

- Blaming tiredness only on age
- Using coffee as your main treatment
- Taking supplements without knowing what you need
- Ignoring sleep quality
- Assuming normal tests explain everything
- Pushing through fatigue without understanding it
- Believing every health claim online

Chapter Summary

Many myths surround tiredness. Some people blame age, sleep, stress, or lack of vitamins too quickly. Others assume normal tests mean nothing is wrong or that coffee and willpower are enough. In reality, fatigue may have many causes, and the right approach is careful observation, proper evaluation, targeted treatment, and steady lifestyle support.

Action Plan

- Identify which fatigue myths you may have believed
- Replace quick assumptions with careful observation
- Review your sleep, medicines, stress, nutrition, and activity
- Avoid random supplements or extreme programs
- Seek medical care when fatigue persists, worsens, or affects daily life
- Choose evidence, not marketing
- Keep looking for the real pattern

Looking Ahead

You now understand the major causes, warning signs, evaluation, treatment, and myths surrounding tiredness.

In the final chapters, we will bring everything together and focus on moving forward with clarity, patience, and confidence.

CHAPTER 21: Moving Forward: Regaining Control of Your Energy

From Confusion to Clarity

When you feel tired all the time, life can begin to feel uncertain.

You may not know whether to rest, exercise, see a doctor, take vitamins, change your sleep, or simply wait. You may try one thing, feel a little better, then slide back again. Over time, tiredness can make you feel as if you are losing control of your own body.

This book was written to change that.

You now know that tiredness is not one single problem. It is a signal. It may come from sleep, stress, nutrition, hormones, chronic disease, infection, medications, emotional strain, inactivity, or several causes at the same time.

Once you understand that, you no longer have to guess blindly.

You can move forward with a plan.

Begin by Listening to Your Body

The first step is not panic. It is attention.

Ask yourself:

When did my tiredness begin?
What has changed in my life?
What makes it better?
What makes it worse?
Do I feel sleepy, weak, breathless, foggy, or emotionally drained?
Are there warning signs?

Your body often gives clues before it gives clear answers.

Listening carefully is not fear. It is wisdom.

Focus on What You Can Control

Fatigue can feel overwhelming if you try to solve everything at once.

Instead, begin with what you can control.

You can improve your sleep routine.
You can eat more regularly.
You can drink water.
You can reduce late caffeine.
You can move gently.
You can review your medicines.
You can ask for help when stress is too heavy.
You can make an appointment when symptoms persist.

These steps may seem small, but they create direction.

And direction creates hope.

Work with Your Doctor

Persistent fatigue is best approached as a partnership.

Your doctor brings medical knowledge, experience, examination, and testing. You bring the story of your body, your habits, your symptoms, your fears, and your daily reality.

Both are needed.

Be honest about sleep, mood, alcohol, caffeine, supplements, stress, medications, pain, bleeding, weight changes, and daily function. These details are not embarrassing. They are useful.

A good diagnosis often begins with a good conversation.

Do Not Demand Perfection from Yourself

Many tired people are already hard on themselves.

They feel guilty for resting. They feel frustrated when they cannot do what they used to do. They compare themselves to others. They think they should be stronger.

But recovery does not come from self-blame.

It comes from steady correction.

One better night of sleep.
One short walk.
One balanced meal.
One honest doctor visit.
One medicine review.
One small boundary with stress.

These are not small victories. They are the foundation of change.

Measure Progress in Trends

Fatigue recovery is rarely a straight line.

You may have better days and worse days. That is normal. Do not judge your recovery by one difficult morning.

Look at trends.

Are you waking a little more refreshed?
Are you thinking more clearly?
Are you needing fewer naps?
Are you walking a little farther?
Are you using less caffeine?
Are you recovering faster after activity?

Progress often appears quietly before it becomes obvious.

Rebuild Confidence Slowly

Constant tiredness can shrink confidence.

A person may stop making plans because they fear they will not have energy. They may avoid travel, exercise, social events, or even ordinary errands. Slowly, life becomes smaller.

One goal of recovery is to rebuild trust in your body.

Start with activities you can manage. Repeat them. Increase gradually. Let success build confidence.

You do not need to return to everything at once.

You only need to begin.

A Patient Example

A 64-year-old man feels tired for months. He worries that he is simply getting old.

After reading and reflecting, he begins tracking his symptoms. He notices poor sleep, late caffeine, reduced walking, and morning fatigue. He sees his doctor and also learns that his blood sugar is high.

His recovery is not instant.

He improves his sleep routine, reduces caffeine, begins walking slowly, follows treatment for blood sugar, and returns for follow-up.

Three months later, he is not perfect, but he feels better. More importantly, he no longer feels helpless.

He has a plan.

Doctor's Pearl

The goal is not just to reduce fatigue.

The goal is to return to life with more strength, clarity, confidence, and hope.

Common Mistakes to Avoid

- Waiting for a perfect solution before starting
- Giving up after one bad day
- Comparing your recovery with someone else's

- Ignoring small improvements
- Hiding important symptoms from your doctor
- Stopping follow-up too soon
- Believing that slow progress means failure

Chapter Summary

Moving forward begins with clarity. Tiredness is a signal that deserves attention, not fear. Recovery often requires careful observation, lifestyle correction, medical evaluation when needed, and patience. Progress may be gradual, but small steps can rebuild energy, confidence, and daily function. The more you understand your body, the less helpless you feel.

Action Plan

- Listen to your body without panic
- Write down your fatigue pattern
- Focus on controllable habits first
- Review sleep, food, hydration, movement, stress, and medicines
- Work honestly with your doctor
- Measure progress over weeks, not days
- Celebrate small improvements
- Continue follow-up if fatigue persists or changes

Looking Ahead

You have now learned how to understand tiredness, recognize warning signs, identify common causes, seek proper evaluation, and begin recovery.

In the final chapter, we will bring the whole message together and leave you with a clear, steady path to take back your energy and your life.

CHAPTER 22: A Final Word: Take Back Your Energy

You Are Not Alone

If you are tired all the time, you may feel alone.

You may feel that others do not fully understand what you are going through. You may look normal from the outside, but inside you may feel drained, foggy, heavy, and discouraged.

Persistent tiredness can quietly affect your confidence. It can make you question your body. It can make you avoid plans, cancel activities, and slowly accept a smaller life.

But you do not have to accept constant tiredness as your new normal.

There is a path forward.

Tiredness Is a Message

The most important message of this book is simple:

Tiredness is not weakness.
Tiredness is information.

Your body may be telling you that something is out of balance. Sometimes the reason is simple. Sometimes it is medical. Sometimes it is emotional. Often, it is a combination of several factors.

The answer is not panic.
The answer is not blame.
The answer is careful attention.

Listen to the symptom. Look for the pattern. Take the next wise step.

What You Now Understand

You now know that tiredness can have many causes.

It may come from poor sleep, sleep apnea, stress, depression, anxiety, anemia, vitamin deficiency, thyroid disease, diabetes, chronic illness, infection, medications, alcohol, caffeine, inactivity, or burnout.

You also know that tiredness should be described clearly.

Are you sleepy?
Are you weak?
Are you breathless?
Are you mentally foggy?
Are you emotionally exhausted?
Do you feel worse after activity?

The clearer your description, the better your care.

Do Not Ignore Warning Signs

Most fatigue is not an emergency, but warning signs matter.

Chest pain, severe shortness of breath, fainting, unexplained weight loss, fever, night sweats, bleeding, black stools, confusion, new neurological symptoms, or severe weakness should not be ignored.

These symptoms deserve prompt medical attention.

Respecting warning signs is not fear. It is wisdom.

Return to the Foundations

The body needs basic support every day.

Good sleep.
Steady meals.
Water.
Gentle movement.
Stress recovery.
Medication review.
Medical care when needed.

These steps may look simple, but they are powerful when practiced consistently.

Do not underestimate ordinary habits. Much of health is built quietly, day after day.

Be Patient with Recovery

Energy often returns gradually.

Some people improve quickly once the cause is treated. Others need more time, especially when fatigue has been present for months or is related to chronic illness, Long COVID, depression, burnout, or deconditioning.

Do not judge your recovery by one bad day.

Look for direction. Look for small gains. Look for better mornings, clearer thinking, longer walks, fewer crashes, and more confidence.

Small progress is still progress.

Work with Your Doctor

You do not need to solve everything alone.

Bring your doctor your story, your symptom pattern, your medicine list, your sleep diary, and your concerns. Be honest about stress, mood, alcohol, caffeine, sleep, supplements, pain, bleeding, and daily function.

A good doctor-patient partnership is one of the strongest tools in fatigue recovery.

Doctor's Pearl

The goal is not simply to feel less tired.

The goal is to live better.

To think more clearly. To move more freely. To work more safely. To enjoy family more fully. To feel more like yourself again.

Common Mistakes to Avoid

- Accepting constant tiredness as normal
- Blaming yourself
- Depending only on caffeine
- Taking random supplements instead of finding the cause

- Ignoring warning signs
- Giving up after slow progress
- Avoiding follow-up when symptoms continue

Final Summary

Tiredness is common, but it should not be dismissed. It may be caused by lifestyle habits, poor sleep, emotional stress, nutritional deficiencies, hormonal problems, chronic diseases, infections, medicines, or several causes together. The best approach is careful observation, proper medical evaluation when needed, targeted treatment, and steady daily habits that support recovery.

Final Action Plan

- Listen to your body
- Describe your tiredness clearly
- Track your sleep, symptoms, medicines, and daily habits
- Watch for warning signs
- Strengthen sleep, nutrition, hydration, movement, and stress recovery
- Review medicines and supplements with your doctor
- Seek medical care when fatigue persists, worsens, or affects daily life
- Stay patient and consistent

A Closing Thought

Energy is not only the ability to stay awake.

Energy is the ability to live with clarity, strength, confidence, and purpose.

If you are tired all the time, do not ignore it. Do not fear it blindly. Do not blame yourself.

Begin with one step.

Listen. Observe. Seek help when needed. Correct what can be corrected. Support your body daily.

You may not regain everything overnight, but you can begin moving in the right direction.

And sometimes, that first steady step is where healing truly begins.

APPENDIX 1: A Practical Self-Assessment Checklist

Start Here: Understand Your Pattern Clearly

Before you try to fix tiredness, take a few minutes to understand it.

This simple checklist helps you organize your symptoms in a way that is useful for both you and your doctor.

Do not rush. Answer honestly.

Your Tiredness Pattern

- When did your tiredness begin?
- Did it start suddenly or gradually?
- Is it getting better, worse, or staying the same?
- Do you feel tired all day or at specific times?
- Do you wake up refreshed or tired?

Type of Tiredness

- Do you feel sleepy during the day?
- Do you feel physically drained?
- Do you feel weak in your muscles?
- Do you feel mentally foggy or slow?
- Do you feel emotionally exhausted or unmotivated?

Sleep Assessment

- What time do you go to bed?
- What time do you wake up?

- Do you wake up during the night?
- Do you snore loudly?
- Has anyone noticed you stop breathing during sleep?
- Do you wake up with a headache or dry mouth?
- Do you nap during the day?

Daily Routine and Habits

- Do you have a regular wake-up time?
- Do you eat regular meals?
- Do you drink enough water?
- How much caffeine do you take, and when?
- Do you use alcohol, especially in the evening?
- How active are you during the day?

Stress and Emotional Health

- Are you under ongoing stress?
- Do you feel anxious or worried frequently?
- Do you feel low, sad, or uninterested in things?
- Do you feel overwhelmed or burned out?
- Are you sleeping poorly because of worry?

Medical Symptoms

- Have you noticed weight loss or weight gain?
- Do you feel short of breath with activity?
- Do you have chest discomfort or palpitations?
- Do you feel dizzy or faint?
- Do you have fever or night sweats?
- Have you noticed bleeding, black stools, or heavy periods?
- Do you have numbness, tingling, or weakness?
- Have you had a recent infection?

Medications and Substances

- List all prescription medicines
- List all over-the-counter medicines
- List vitamins and supplements
- Note any recent changes in dose or new medicines
- How much alcohol do you drink?
- How much caffeine do you use?

How Tiredness Affects Your Life

- Does it affect your work?
- Does it affect your concentration?
- Does it affect your mood?
- Does it affect your relationships?
- Does it affect your safety, such as driving?

Doctor's Pearl

A clear description is often the first step toward a clear diagnosis.

Bring this checklist to your doctor. It can save time and improve the quality of your care.

APPENDIX 2: Simple Daily Energy Log

Track for 7–14 Days

Use this log to observe patterns. You do not need to write long sentences. Short notes are enough.

Each Day, Record:

Sleep:

- Bedtime
- Wake time
- Number of awakenings
- How you felt on waking (refreshed or tired)

Daytime Energy:

- Morning energy (good / fair / poor)
- Afternoon energy (good / fair / poor)
- Evening energy (good / fair / poor)

Activity:

- Type of activity (walking, work, chores)
- Duration
- Did activity improve or worsen fatigue?

Food and Drink:

- Meals (regular or skipped)
- Caffeine (amount and time)
- Alcohol (if any)
- Water intake

Symptoms:

- Shortness of breath
- Dizziness
- Pain
- Mood changes
- Brain fog
- Any unusual symptoms

Why This Matters

Patterns often appear only when you write things down.

You may notice:

- Poor sleep before bad days
- Late caffeine affecting sleep
- Activity helping or worsening fatigue
- Mood changes affecting energy

This information is very useful for your doctor.

APPENDIX 3: When to Seek Medical Help Urgently

Do Not Delay Care If You Have:

- Chest pain or pressure
- Severe shortness of breath
- Fainting or near-fainting
- Black stools or vomiting blood
- Unexplained weight loss
- Fever or night sweats
- Confusion or difficulty speaking
- New weakness on one side of the body
- Severe dizziness
- Thoughts of self-harm

These symptoms may not always mean a serious condition, but they require prompt medical evaluation.

APPENDIX 4: A Simple 30-Day Energy Reset Plan

Week 1: Awareness

- Track your sleep, energy, food, caffeine, and activity
- Identify patterns
- Note warning signs if present

Week 2: Sleep Reset

- Fix a consistent wake-up time
- Reduce caffeine after lunch
- Avoid alcohol near bedtime
- Create a calm evening routine

Week 3: Fuel and Movement

- Eat regular meals with protein
- Drink water regularly
- Begin gentle activity (such as 10–15 minutes of walking daily if safe)

Week 4: Review and Adjust

- Review what improved
- Identify what still needs attention
- Decide if medical evaluation is needed
- Continue helpful habits

Doctor's Pearl

You do not need a perfect plan.

You need a plan you can follow.

FINAL THOUGHT

These appendixes are not meant to overwhelm you.

They are meant to guide you.

Use them step by step. Take your time. Be consistent.

Clarity comes first. Improvement follows.

Thank You and Please Review the Book

Thank you for taking the time to read this book. I sincerely hope it has helped you understand your health a little more clearly and has given you practical, everyday steps you can follow with confidence. If you found this book helpful, **I would truly appreciate it if you could leave a brief and honest review.** Even a few lines sharing your experience can make a meaningful difference. Your feedback helps other readers find reliable, trustworthy health information and supports them in making better decisions for themselves and their families.

Warm regards,

Dr Prabhat Das

Continue your Healthcare Journey with these Books

Good health is a journey, not a single step. It is not achieved in one day or with one book. That is why I created the "Better Health with Dr Das Series", with each book addressing a different common condition. If you would like easy, practical guidance on other everyday health concerns, you may wish to explore the rest of books in this series.

Books in this series:

- Better Health starts Here: A Doctor's Guide to Staying Healthy After 40
- A Doctor's Easy Guide to Understanding & Managing OBESITY
- Doctor, What DIET Is Best for Me?
- Doctor, Why Can't I Lose Weight? A Doctor's Guide to Safe & Sustainable Weight Loss)
- A Doctor's Easy Guide to GLP-1 for Obesity
- A Doctor's Easy Guide to Understanding & Managing HIGH BLOOD PRESSURE
- A Doctor's Guide to Living Well With DIABETES
- A Doctor's Guide to Understanding & Managing THYROID DISEASES
- A Doctor's Guide to Understanding & Managing HIGH CHOLESTEROL
- A Doctor's Practical Guide to HEART HEALTH After 40: How to Protect Your Heart & Live Longer
- A Doctor's Guide to Healing & Reversing FATTY LIVER DISEASE: Simple, Natural & Science-Based Steps to Reduce Liver Fat and Prevent Complications

- Control Your ACID REFLUX, HEARTBURN & GERD: A Doctor's Practical Guide that Works
- Live Comfortably with IRRITABLE BOWEL SYNDROME: A Doctor's Practical Guide to Understanding & Managing IBS
- A Doctor's Practical Guide to Understanding & Managing GALLBLADDER STONES & OTHER PROBLEMS
- Take Control of COPD: A Doctor's Practical Guide to Better Breathing
- Living Better with ASTHMA: A Doctor's Practical Guide to Asthma Control
- SLEEP APNEA, INSOMNIA & OTHER SLEEP DISORDERS: A Doctor's Practical Guide to Better Sleep & Better Health
- Protect Your KIDNEYS: A Doctor's Practical Guide to Kidney Health & Prevention
- PROSTATE HEALTH: A Doctor's Practical Guide to Early Detection & Care
- ARTHRITIS: A Doctor's Practical Guide to Pain Control & Mobility
- STROKE: A Doctor's Practical Guide to Prevention & Early detection
- HEART ATTACK: A Doctor's Practical Guide to Prevention & Early detection
- CANCER: A Doctor's Practical Guide to Prevention & Early detection
- BACK PAIN: A Doctor's Practical Guide to Fixing Step by Step
- COMMON SKIN & HAIR PROBLEMS: A Doctor's Practical Guide to Skin & Hair Care
- DEMENTIA & MEMORY LOSS: A Doctor's Practical Guide to Prevention & Management

- TIRED ALL THE TIME: A Doctor's Practical Guide to Finding the Cause & Rebuilding Your Energy

www.ingramcontent.com/pod-product-compliance
Lightning Source LLC
LaVergne TN
LVHW010320220926
848484LV00004BB/808
9781971672793